CODE BLUE

Tales From the Emergency Room

Volume 7

JEFFREY CHAMBERS, M.D.

FREE REIGN

ISBN 13: 979-8-89234-068-7

Free Reign Publishing, LLC
San Diego, CA

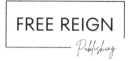

Contents

Introduction

In the series, *Code Blue: Tales from the Emergency Room,* Dr. Chambers offers a gripping behind-the-scenes look into the world of emergency medicine. With vivid, heart-pounding narratives, he draws us into the intense, unpredictable world of the ER, where split-second decisions can mean the difference between life and death.

This isn't just a book about medicine. It's about resilience and vulnerability, about the fine line between hope and despair. It's about the moments of triumph and tragedy that medical professionals witness daily, moments that are often shielded from the public's eye. Dr. Chambers, with unflinching honesty, gives voice to the unsung heroes – nurses, technicians, paramedics, and of course, the patients themselves – who populate the ER.

As you turn these pages, you'll venture on a roller-coaster ride of emotions, from the heartache of a family saying their final goodbyes, to the joyous relief of a child's life saved against all odds. These tales will make you question, reflect, and marvel at the boundless spirit of humanity.

Code Blue is more than just a collection of stories; it's a tribute to the chaotic, beautiful, and profoundly human world of the emergency room. Whether you're a medical professional, a patient, or simply a curious reader, Dr. Chambers welcomes you to step through those sliding glass doors, to witness the raw, undiluted reality of life in the ER.

Prepare to be moved, inspired, and forever changed.

Chapter 1
SACROCOCCYGEAL TERATOMA

I HAVE ENCOUNTERED countless cases that tested my medical expertise and emotional endurance. Among these, one particular case involving a patient with a sacrococcygeal teratoma stands out. The journey from diagnosis to treatment, and the eventual outcome, was a profound experience that left a lasting impact on my career and personal life.

The patient, a newborn, was brought to our hospital by concerned parents who had noticed a peculiar mass at the base of the baby's spine. During the initial examination, I observed a large, protruding mass in the sacrococcygeal region. The mass was firm to the touch and had a heterogeneous consistency. Given the location and nature of the mass, I immediately suspected a sacrococcygeal teratoma, a rare tumor that can arise from the coccyx.

To confirm the diagnosis, we performed a series of diagnostic tests. An ultrasound was the first step, revealing a complex mass with cystic and solid components. This finding was consistent with a teratoma, but we needed more detailed imaging to assess the extent of the tumor and its involvement with surrounding structures. A subsequent MRI provided a clearer picture, showing a well-defined mass extending from the sacrum to the coccyx, with both internal and external components. The tumor appeared to be compressing adjacent tissues but had not invaded any vital organs, which was a hopeful sign.

With the diagnosis confirmed, the next step was to determine the best course of treatment. Sacrococcygeal teratomas can range from benign to malignant, and the treatment approach would depend heavily on the tumor's pathology. We performed a biopsy, carefully obtaining a sample of the tumor tissue. The pathology report indicated that the teratoma was predominantly mature, meaning it was composed of differentiated tissues from multiple germ layers. However, there were areas of immature tissue, suggesting a risk of malignancy.

Given the mixed nature of the tumor, we decided

to proceed with surgical resection as the primary treatment. The goal was to remove the entire tumor, including the coccyx, to minimize the risk of recurrence. The surgery was scheduled promptly, considering the patient's age and the potential complications of delaying treatment.

The surgical team, comprising experienced pediatric surgeons and anesthesiologists, prepared meticulously for the procedure. The patient was placed under general anesthesia, and the surgical field was prepped. An incision was made over the sacrococcygeal region, and the surgeons carefully dissected through layers of tissue to reach the tumor. The mass was meticulously separated from surrounding structures, taking great care to avoid damaging nearby nerves and blood vessels.

As the surgeons worked, it became evident that the tumor was larger and more complex than initially anticipated. It extended deeper into the pelvis, requiring precise and delicate maneuvers to ensure complete removal. Despite the challenges, the surgical team persevered, and after several hours, they successfully excised the entire tumor along with the coccyx.

The patient was then transferred to the neonatal intensive care unit (NICU) for post-operative care. The immediate post-surgical period was critical, as we monitored for any signs of complications such as infection, bleeding, or issues with wound healing. The patient showed remarkable fortitude, gradually stabilizing over the following days.

With the tumor removed, our focus shifted to the patient's recovery and ongoing monitoring. The pathology report on the resected tumor confirmed that while most of the tissue was mature, there were indeed areas of immaturity. This finding necessitated regular follow-up to detect any signs of recurrence or malignant transformation. We initiated a comprehensive surveillance plan, including periodic imaging studies and tumor marker evaluations.

The patient's recovery in the NICU was closely supervised by a multidisciplinary team. Nutritional support, pain management, and physical therapy were integral parts of the care plan. The incision site healed without major complications, and the patient gradually regained strength and activity levels. However, the journey was far from over, as the long-term prognosis for sacrococcygeal teratoma can be unpredictable.

In the ensuing months, the patient returned for scheduled follow-up visits. Each visit involved a thorough physical examination, imaging studies such as MRI or ultrasound, and blood tests to measure levels of alpha-fetoprotein (AFP), a marker often elevated in cases of germ cell tumors. The initial post-operative scans were encouraging, showing no evidence of residual or recurrent tumor.

Despite the favorable early results, the inherent unpredictability of sacrococcygeal teratomas kept us vigilant. The patient continued to grow and develop, hitting typical milestones, but the specter of recurrence lingered. We educated the parents on signs to watch for, emphasizing the importance of regular check-ups and adherence to the follow-up schedule.

Around a year post-surgery, during a routine follow-up, we detected a slight increase in AFP levels. Although not alarmingly high, this warranted further investigation. An MRI was performed, revealing a small, suspicious area near the previous tumor site. The finding was subtle, but given the history, we opted for a cautious approach.

A second surgery was scheduled to explore and, if necessary, excise any residual tumor. The procedure was less extensive than the initial surgery, but equally critical. The surgeons found a small nodule, which they excised and sent for pathology. The pathology report confirmed that the nodule was an immature teratoma, indicating a potential for malignant transformation if left untreated.

The patient recovered well from the second surgery,

and subsequent follow-up visits showed stable AFP levels and no further signs of recurrence. We remained cautiously optimistic, but the need for ongoing surveillance was clear. The patient continued to undergo regular imaging and blood tests, a routine that became a part of their life.

As the years passed, the patient grew into a healthy child, showing no signs of developmental delays or physical impairments. The regular follow-ups became less frequent but continued to be a part of their health-care regimen. The risk of recurrence diminishes with time, but it never completely disappears, especially with a history of immature teratoma.

Reflecting on this case, I am reminded of the complexity and unpredictability of medical practice. The patient's journey from diagnosis to treatment and recovery was a testament to the advances in pediatric oncology and surgery. It also highlighted the impor-tance of early detection, multidisciplinary care, and long-term monitoring in managing rare and chal-lenging conditions like sacrococcygeal teratoma.

Throughout the process, the patient's strength and the unwavering support of their family were crucial. While we as medical professionals provided the exper-tise and care, the patient's indomitable spirit played an equally important role in their recovery. This case reinforced my belief in the resilience of the human body and the profound impact of comprehensive medical care.

As a physician, I have encountered many challenging cases, but this patient's journey remains etched in my memory. It serves as a reminder of the delicate balance between medical science and the human elements of care, underscoring the importance of empathy, vigilance, and perseverance in the face of uncertainty.

Chapter 2
WEIL SYNDROME

THE SUMMER HAD BEEN UNUSUALLY wet, a fact that hadn't escaped any of us at the small county hospital where I worked. The rain had swollen rivers and flooded fields, creating an ideal breeding ground for pests and pathogens alike. It was in this context that the patient first arrived, presenting with symptoms that seemed, at first, to be nothing more than a particularly nasty case of the flu.

The patient was a middle-aged man, appearing gaunt and weary, his skin pallid beneath a sheen of sweat. He was escorted into my examination room by a concerned relative, who explained that he had been suffering from high fever, chills, and severe headaches for the past few days. His muscles ached, his appetite was nonexistent, and he was barely able to keep any fluids down. As I took his medical history, I learned that he had been working in the fields near the river, which had overflowed several weeks earlier.

My initial suspicion was that he was suffering from leptospirosis, a bacterial infection commonly transmitted through water contaminated with the urine of infected animals. I ordered a battery of tests, including blood cultures and a complete blood count, to confirm my hypothesis. In the meantime, I started him on a regimen of broad-spectrum antibiotics to cover a range of possible bacterial infections, and I admitted him to the hospital for observation and supportive care.

The patient's condition deteriorated rapidly. By the next morning, his fever had spiked to over 104 degrees Fahrenheit, and he was experiencing severe jaundice. His eyes, once a clear blue, had turned a disturbing shade of yellow, and his skin had taken on a similar hue. He was disoriented, slipping in and out of consciousness, and his breathing had become labored.

The blood test results confirmed my worst fears: the patient was suffering from Weil syndrome, a severe form of leptospirosis. This condition can cause liver and kidney failure, meningitis, and respiratory distress, among other complications. The bacteria, Leptospira, had invaded his bloodstream and was wreaking havoc on his organs.

We intensified his treatment immediately. High doses of intravenous penicillin were administered to combat the bacterial infection, and we provided aggressive supportive care to manage his symptoms. His electrolyte balance was dangerously unstable, so we administered fluids and electrolytes intravenously. We monitored his liver and kidney function closely, prepared to initiate dialysis if his kidneys continued to fail. His jaundice suggested significant liver damage, so we consulted with a hepatologist to devise a plan to support his liver function.

The next few days were a harrowing blur of interventions and close monitoring. Despite our best efforts, the patient's condition remained precarious. His liver function tests showed alarming levels of bilirubin and transaminases, indicating severe hepatic injury. His kidneys were not faring much better; his creatinine levels were climbing steadily, a sign that his renal function was deteriorating. We initiated dialysis as his urine output dwindled to almost nothing.

In the midst of all this, we were also fighting to keep his respiratory system functioning. His lungs were filling with fluid, a complication of both the infection and his failing organs. He required supplemental oxygen, and we discussed the possibility of intubation and mechanical ventilation if his condition did not improve.

Throughout this ordeal, the patient's mental state was a rollercoaster. There were moments of lucidity where he seemed to comprehend the gravity of his situation, followed by periods of delirium where he would thrash weakly and mutter incoherently. We administered sedatives sparingly, trying to balance his comfort with the need to keep his vital signs stable.

As the days turned into a week, there were small glimmers of hope. His fever began to subside, and his blood cultures showed a decrease in bacterial load. The antibiotics seemed to be taking effect, and his liver and kidney function showed slight improvements. His jaundice, while still pronounced, began to lessen, and his urine output increased modestly, suggesting that his kidneys were starting to recover.

However, the road to recovery was fraught with setbacks. He developed a secondary bacterial pneumonia, a common complication in patients who are severely ill and bedridden. This required a new round of antibiotics and further strained his already weakened body. He also experienced episodes of sepsis, where the infection would flare up and send his body into a state of shock, requiring emergency interventions to stabilize his blood pressure and organ function.

Through it all, the patient demonstrated an extraordinary capacity to endure. His physical strength waned, but there was a tenacity in his fight against the illness that was palpable. We continued our vigilant care, adjusting treatments as needed and constantly reassessing his progress.

After two weeks of intensive treatment, the patient's condition began to show more consistent signs of improvement. His liver and kidney function, while still impaired, stabilized enough that we could reduce the frequency of dialysis sessions. His jaundice gradually faded, and his energy levels began to return. He was able to sit up in bed and eat small amounts of food, a significant milestone after days of intravenous nutrition.

The pneumonia responded well to the antibiotics, and his respiratory function improved enough that we could wean him off supplemental oxygen. His mental clarity returned, and he was able to engage in conversations, though they were often brief and tiring for him.

As the patient continued to recover, we shifted our focus to rehabilitation. His muscles had atrophied from weeks of bed rest, and he required physical therapy to regain his strength and mobility. This was a slow and painstaking process, but he approached it with the same determination that had carried him through the worst of his illness.

By the time he was ready to be discharged from the hospital, the patient was a shadow of the man who had first walked into my examination room. He had lost a significant amount of weight, and his skin still bore the yellowish tinge of jaundice, though it was much improved. His kidneys were functioning well enough that he no longer required dialysis, and his liver enzymes had returned to near-normal levels.

The recovery process continued at home, with regular follow-up appointments to monitor his progress and adjust his treatment as needed. He faced months of physical therapy and had to adhere to a strict regimen of medications to support his liver and kidney function. There were also lifestyle changes to consider, such as avoiding activities that could expose him to leptospirosis in the future.

Reflecting on the patient's journey, I was struck by the profound impact of timely and aggressive medical intervention. Without the antibiotics, supportive care, and constant monitoring, his chances of survival would have been slim. It was a testament to the advances in medical science and the dedication of the healthcare team that he was able to make such a remarkable recovery.

In the end, the patient's story was one of triumph over a life-threatening illness. His journey through the depths of Weil syndrome to the gradual restoration of his health was a powerful reminder of the fragility and resilience of the human body. It also underscored the importance of early diagnosis and treatment in managing severe infections and preventing long-term complications.

As a doctor, it was a privilege to be part of his recovery, to witness his courage, and to contribute to his healing. The experience reaffirmed my commitment to providing compassionate and comprehensive care to all my patients, knowing that each case, no matter how challenging, holds the potential for recovery and renewal.

Chapter 3
BACHMANN-BUPP SYNDROME

I FIRST ENCOUNTERED the patient in the bustling chaos of the emergency room. It was a typical Tuesday night, filled with the usual rush of traumas and minor ailments. The patient had been brought in by concerned family members, and his symptoms were perplexing. He had been experiencing severe muscle weakness, difficulty swallowing, and unexplained weight loss. His condition had deteriorated rapidly over the past few weeks, and his family was desperate for answers.

As I examined him, I noted the telltale signs of muscle atrophy. His once-robust frame had withered, leaving him frail and gaunt. His speech was slurred, and he struggled to articulate his words. These symptoms pointed towards a neuromuscular disorder, but the rapid progression and severity were unusual. I ordered a battery of tests, including blood work, electromyography, and a muscle biopsy, to narrow down the possibilities.

The initial results were inconclusive. His blood work showed elevated levels of creatine kinase, indicating muscle damage, but there was no clear indication of an inflammatory or autoimmune process. The electromyography revealed abnormal electrical activity in his muscles, consistent with a myopathy, but it did not provide a definitive diagnosis. The muscle biopsy, however, was more revealing. The histological examination showed a pattern of vacuolar myopathy with rimmed vacuoles, a hallmark of Bachmann-Bupp Syndrome.

Bachmann-Bupp Syndrome is a rare genetic disorder characterized by progressive muscle weakness and wasting. It is caused by mutations in the VCP gene, which plays a crucial role in protein homeostasis and the degradation of misfolded proteins. The syndrome can present with a wide range of symptoms, including muscle weakness, dysphagia, respiratory insufficiency, and cardiomyopathy. Given the patient's symptoms and the biopsy findings, the diagnosis was clear.

Breaking the news to the patient and his family was challenging. Bachmann-Bupp Syndrome is a progressive and debilitating condition, and there is no cure. The prognosis varies, but many patients experience a gradual decline in muscle function and respiratory capacity. I explained the nature of the disease, the expected progression, and the available treatment options. Our focus would be on managing symptoms and maintaining his quality of life for as long as possible.

The cornerstone of treatment for Bachmann-Bupp Syndrome is supportive care. We started the patient on a regimen of physical therapy to preserve his remaining muscle strength and improve his mobility. Occupational therapy helped him adapt to his daily activities and maintain his independence. Speech therapy was essential for addressing his dysphagia and ensuring he could continue to eat and drink safely. Additionally, we arranged for respiratory therapy to monitor and support his breathing.

Medications played a role in managing his symptoms as well. We prescribed corticosteroids to reduce muscle inflammation and slow the progression of muscle weakness. Immunosuppressive drugs were considered, but their efficacy in treating Bachmann-Bupp Syndrome is uncertain, and the potential side effects are significant. We opted for a conservative approach, focusing on symptomatic relief rather than aggressive immunosuppression.

As the weeks turned into months, the patient's condition stabilized. The physical therapy regimen helped him regain some of his lost strength, and he became more adept at using assistive devices to aid his mobility. He faced his daily challenges with remarkable determination, adapting to his new reality with a quiet fortitude. His family remained a constant source of support, helping him navigate the complexities of his treatment and providing emotional encouragement.

Despite our best efforts, the progressive nature of Bachmann-Bupp Syndrome became increasingly evident. The patient's muscle weakness continued to advance, and he began to experience more frequent episodes of respiratory difficulty. We closely monitored his lung function, and when his respiratory capacity declined below a critical threshold, we discussed the option of non-invasive ventilation to support his breathing at night.

The introduction of non-invasive ventilation was a turning point. The patient initially resisted the idea, finding the mask cumbersome and uncomfortable. However, as he experienced the benefits of improved sleep quality and reduced daytime fatigue, he became more accepting of the treatment. The ventilation provided much-needed support for his weakening respiratory muscles, allowing him to maintain a semblance of normalcy in his daily life.

As a physician, witnessing the gradual decline of a patient with a progressive disease is always heart-wrenching. The patient's courage in the face of adversity was inspiring, but it was clear that his condition was taking a toll on him physically and emotionally. He struggled with feelings of frustration and helplessness as his body continued to betray him. The psychological impact of his illness was as significant as the physical symptoms, and we provided counseling and support to help him cope with the emotional burden.

In the latter stages of his illness, the patient's condition deteriorated more rapidly. His respiratory function declined further, and he began to experience frequent infections due to his weakened immune system. Each bout of pneumonia or bronchitis left him more debilitated, and his ability to recover diminished with each episode. We managed these complications with antibiotics and supportive care, but it was clear that his body was losing the battle.

The decision to transition to palliative care was a difficult but necessary one. The focus shifted from prolonging life to ensuring comfort and dignity in his final days. We worked closely with a palliative care team to manage his symptoms, providing pain relief, respiratory support, and emotional comfort. The patient and his family were involved in every step of the decision-making process, ensuring that his wishes were respected and that he received the best possible care.

The end came quietly one evening. The patient passed away surrounded by his loved ones, his suffering finally at an end. The journey from diagnosis to his final moments had been a challenging and emotional one for everyone involved. As a doctor, it was a reminder of the limits of medicine and the importance of compassionate care. While we could not cure his disease, we had provided him with the best possible quality of life and supported him and his family through their darkest times.

Reflecting on the patient's journey, I was struck by the strength of the human spirit in the face of relentless adversity. His determination to live each day to the fullest, despite the limitations imposed by his illness, was a testament to his indomitable will. His family's unwavering support and love were equally remarkable, providing a foundation of strength and comfort throughout his illness.

The experience of treating the patient with Bach-mann-Bupp Syndrome left an indelible mark on me. It underscored the importance of a holistic approach to medicine, where the focus is not just on the disease but on the individual and their overall well-being. It reinforced the value of interdisciplinary care, where different specialties come together to address the multifaceted challenges of complex diseases.

In the months following the patient's passing, I continued to think about the lessons learned from his case. His journey had highlighted the need for ongoing research and advancements in the treatment of rare genetic disorders. While we had done our best with the available knowledge and resources, there was a pressing need for better therapies and a deeper understanding of the underlying mechanisms of diseases like Bachmann-Bupp Syndrome.

The patient's case also emphasized the importance of empathy and communication in medical practice. Building a strong, trusting relationship with patients and their families is crucial, especially when dealing with life-altering diagnoses. Clear, compassionate communication can help patients and their loved ones navigate the uncertainties and challenges of their illness, providing them with a sense of control and understanding.

As I continued my work, I carried the memory of the patient with me. His story served as a reminder of the profound impact that healthcare providers can have on the lives of their patients. It reinforced my commitment to providing compassionate, patient-centered care and to advocating for advancements in the treatment of rare and complex diseases.

In the end, the patient's journey was one of courage, endurance, and unwavering spirit. Despite the challenges and suffering, he faced his illness with dignity and grace. His legacy lived on in the hearts of those who knew him and in the lessons he imparted to those of us who had the privilege of caring for him.

Chapter 4
DE BARSY SYNDROME

I HAD BEEN A PRACTICING pediatrician for over a decade when the patient first came to my attention. The family had been referred to me by a concerned general practitioner who had noticed the child's unusual physical characteristics and developmental delays. As soon as the patient walked into my office, escorted by their anxious parents, I felt an immediate tug of concern. The child, no older than four, had a strikingly unique appearance that was hard to overlook. They had an aged face with deep-set eyes, a prominent forehead, and a receding jaw. These were telltale signs of De Barsy Syndrome, a rare genetic disorder that I had only read about in medical literature.

The initial consultation was thorough. I meticulously documented the patient's medical history, noting that the parents had first noticed developmental delays when the child was around one year old. They had initially thought the delays were minor, but as time passed, it became evident that something was amiss. The patient had difficulty with basic motor skills, and their cognitive development lagged significantly behind their peers. The general practitioner had been at a loss, and I could see why.

I conducted a full physical examination, paying close attention to the patient's skin, which was unusually lax and wrinkled for someone so young. I also noted the presence of cataracts in both eyes, a condition that is not only rare in children but also indicative of systemic issues. The combination of these physical characteristics and developmental delays strongly suggested De Barsy Syndrome. However, diagnosing such a rare condition required more than clinical observation; it required genetic testing to confirm.

I ordered a series of tests, including a comprehensive metabolic panel, an MRI of the brain, and a genetic panel. The genetic test was the most critical, as it would allow us to identify any mutations in the PYCR1 or ALDH18A1 genes, which are commonly associated with De Barsy Syndrome. The wait for results was excruciating for the family, but it was necessary to ensure an accurate diagnosis.

While we awaited the genetic test results, I explained to the parents what De Barsy Syndrome entailed. It is an autosomal recessive disorder, meaning both parents must carry the defective gene for their child to be affected. The syndrome is characterized by progeroid features, joint laxity, and developmental delays, among other symptoms. I could see the fear and confusion in their eyes as they absorbed the information. It was a lot to take in, but I assured them that we would take this one step at a time.

The test results confirmed my suspicions. The patient had mutations in both copies of the PYCR1 gene. It was a definitive diagnosis of De Barsy Syndrome. The parents were devastated, and I felt a profound sense of sorrow for them. Their child faced a lifetime of challenges, and there was no cure for this condition. Our focus would be on managing symptoms and improving the patient's quality of life as much as possible.

Treatment began immediately. The first step was to address the cataracts, as they were already affecting the patient's vision. I referred the family to a pediatric ophthalmologist who specialized in congenital cataract removal. The surgery was successful, and the patient's vision improved significantly, though they would still need corrective lenses.

Next, we tackled the joint laxity and motor skill delays. I referred the patient to a pediatric physical therapist who developed a customized plan to help improve strength and coordination. The therapy sessions were intensive and required a great deal of patience and dedication from both the patient and their parents. Over time, we saw some improvement, but progress was slow and painstaking.

Cognitively, the patient required special education services. I worked closely with the family to get them in touch with a local early intervention program that specialized in developmental delays. The patient received individualized education plans that focused on enhancing cognitive abilities and social skills. The teachers and therapists were compassionate and dedicated, providing a supportive environment for the patient to learn and grow.

Medically, we had to monitor the patient closely for other potential complications. Children with De Barsy Syndrome are at increased risk for various health issues, including cardiovascular problems, respiratory difficulties, and metabolic imbalances. Regular check-ups and screenings became a routine part of the patient's life. Each visit was an opportunity to catch any emerging issues early and address them promptly.

The patient's condition required a multidisciplinary

approach. I coordinated with a team of specialists, including geneticists, cardiologists, pulmonologists, and nutritionists, to ensure comprehensive care. Communication among the team was crucial, as any changes in the patient's health could have widespread implications. The family was actively involved in every step of the process, becoming well-versed in their child's condition and the necessary treatments.

Despite our best efforts, the road was fraught with challenges. There were periods of relative stability, but they were often followed by setbacks. The patient developed scoliosis, a common complication in De Barsy Syndrome, and had to wear a back brace to prevent further curvature of the spine. This was uncomfortable and restricting, but necessary to maintain their mobility.

As the patient grew older, managing the condition became increasingly complex. The physical and cognitive gaps between them and their peers widened, leading to social isolation and emotional distress. I referred the family to a child psychologist who specialized in chronic illness and developmental disorders. Therapy provided a safe space for the patient to express their feelings and learn coping strategies.

One of the most heartbreaking aspects of De Barsy Syndrome is its progressive nature. Despite early interventions and continuous care, the patient's condition gradually worsened. By the time they reached adolescence, they were experiencing more severe health issues. Respiratory problems became more frequent, and they had to be hospitalized multiple times for pneumonia and other infections. Their immune system was compromised, making them vulnerable to common illnesses that their body struggled to fight off.

Throughout this period, the family demonstrated an extraordinary level of commitment and fortitude. They became advocates for their child, educating themselves about the syndrome and seeking out the best possible care. They participated in support groups, connecting with other families facing similar challenges, which provided a sense of community and shared understanding.

The decline in the patient's health was relentless. By their late teens, they required more intensive medical support. They were frequently in and out of the hospital, and managing their care became a full-time job for the parents. The patient's spirit, though, remained unbroken. They faced each day with a quiet determination that was truly remarkable.

In their final years, the focus of treatment shifted from aggressive interventions to palliative care. It was clear that the patient's body could no longer withstand the onslaught of complications. Our goal became one of providing comfort and maintaining the best quality of life possible. Pain management, respiratory support, and nutritional care were prioritized.

The end came quietly. The patient passed away in their sleep, surrounded by their family. It was a peaceful passing, free from the pain and struggle that had characterized much of their life. The family was devastated, but they also expressed a profound sense of relief that their child was no longer suffering.

Reflecting on the patient's journey, I was struck by the profound impact they had on everyone around them. Despite the many challenges they faced, the patient's unwavering spirit and the family's steadfast dedication left an indelible mark on me and on the entire medical team. Their story was a testament to the strength of the human spirit in the face of unimaginable adversity.

In the aftermath, I remained in contact with the family. They became advocates for rare genetic disorders, working to raise awareness and funding for research. Their experience highlighted the importance of early diagnosis, comprehensive care, and the need for ongoing support for families dealing with similar conditions.

The patient's life, though brief, had a lasting

impact. Their journey underscored the critical need for research and advancements in genetic disorders. Each case of De Barsy Syndrome is a reminder of the work that still needs to be done, the breakthroughs yet to be achieved, and the lives that hang in the balance.

As a doctor, I was humbled by the experience. It reinforced my commitment to providing compassionate, comprehensive care to all my patients, regardless of the rarity or severity of their condition. The patient's story was a poignant reminder that medicine is not just about curing diseases but also about caring for people, supporting families, and striving to improve the quality of life for those we serve.

Chapter 5
FACTOR XI DEFICIENCY

AS A DOCTOR, I had seen countless patients, each with their unique stories and struggles. Yet, there was one case that would forever stand out in my mind. It was a chilly morning in late November when the patient was brought into the clinic. The patient was a middle-aged individual with a pallor that hinted at more than just a bad night's sleep. The patient complained of frequent nosebleeds and excessive bruising from minor bumps, symptoms that had been persistent for months.

After a thorough physical examination and a detailed medical history review, I decided to order a complete blood count and a coagulation profile. The results were alarming. The patient's partial thromboplastin time (PTT) was significantly prolonged, indicating a problem with the intrinsic pathway of the coagulation cascade. This finding, combined with the patient's symptoms, prompted me to delve deeper into the patient's coagulation status. I ordered a series of specific factor assays to pinpoint the exact deficiency.

The results were conclusive. The patient had Factor XI deficiency, a rare bleeding disorder. Factor XI, an essential component of the blood clotting process, plays a critical role in stabilizing clots and preventing excessive bleeding. Without sufficient levels of this factor, even minor injuries could lead to significant blood loss.

The patient was understandably distressed upon hearing the diagnosis. I explained that Factor XI deficiency, also known as hemophilia C, is a condition that can vary widely in its severity. Some individuals might experience minimal symptoms, while others could face life-threatening bleeding episodes. In this case, the patient's frequent nosebleeds and bruising indicated a more severe manifestation of the disorder.

Our first step in managing the condition was to prevent any potential bleeding episodes. The patient was advised to avoid activities that could lead to injury. Medications that could exacerbate bleeding, such as aspirin and nonsteroidal anti-inflammatory drugs, were strictly prohibited. I also provided the patient with an emergency contact card indicating their condition, which would be crucial in the event of an accident or emergency surgery.

Despite these precautions, the patient soon experienced a significant bleeding episode. A minor fall at home resulted in a large hematoma on the patient's thigh. The bruise was not only painful but also grew alarmingly large within hours. The patient was admitted to the hospital for closer observation and treatment.

In the hospital, we started treatment with fresh frozen plasma (FFP), which contains all the clotting factors, including Factor XI. The patient responded well to the transfusion, and the bleeding was brought under control. However, this episode highlighted the precarious nature of the patient's condition. We needed a more sustainable treatment plan to manage the bleeding risk effectively.

Given the patient's frequent bleeding episodes, we decided to explore the possibility of using antifibrinolytic agents. These medications, such as tranexamic acid, help to stabilize clots by preventing their premature breakdown. The patient was started on a regimen of tranexamic acid, and we closely monitored the response.

The initial results were promising. The patient's bruises healed more quickly, and the frequency of nosebleeds decreased. However, the underlying deficiency remained, and the patient was at constant risk of spontaneous bleeding. We discussed the option of Factor XI concentrate, a more targeted therapy that could potentially offer better control of bleeding. Unfortunately, Factor XI concentrate is not widely available and can be prohibitively expensive.

Despite these challenges, we remained vigilant. Regular follow-up appointments were scheduled to monitor the patient's coagulation status and overall health. Each visit was a reminder of the fragile balance we were trying to maintain. The patient's blood work was closely scrutinized, and adjustments to the treatment regimen were made as needed.

Months turned into years, and the patient adapted to living with the condition. The patient's courage and perseverance were remarkable. Despite the constant threat of bleeding, the patient maintained a positive outlook and adhered to the treatment plan diligently. The antifibrinolytic therapy, combined with careful lifestyle adjustments, allowed the patient to manage the condition reasonably well.

However, living with Factor XI deficiency was not without its complications. The patient experienced several minor bleeding episodes, each a stark reminder of the condition's severity. One particularly challenging episode occurred during a routine dental procedure. Despite taking all necessary precautions, the patient developed significant postoperative bleeding. Another hospital admission and a transfusion of FFP were required to stabilize the situation.

The patient's quality of life was undeniably impacted. Social activities were curtailed, and physical exertion was limited to minimize the risk of injury. The psychological burden of living with a chronic bleeding disorder was immense. The patient often expressed feelings of isolation and frustration, compounded by the constant need for vigilance.

As the years passed, medical advancements offered new hope. Research into gene therapy for hemophilia had made significant strides, and clinical trials were underway. These therapies aimed to introduce functional copies of the defective gene responsible for Factor XI production, potentially offering a long-term solution. However, these treatments were still in the experimental stages and not yet available for widespread use.

The patient's health remained relatively stable until a fateful day in late summer. The patient was involved in a minor car accident. Although the physical injuries were not severe, the impact triggered significant internal bleeding. The patient was rushed to the emergency room, where we quickly initiated treatment with FFP and antifibrinolytic agents.

Despite our best efforts, the bleeding proved difficult to control. The patient's condition deteriorated rapidly, and the bleeding caused a cascade of complications, including hypovolemic shock. Intensive care measures were implemented, but the severity of the bleeding overwhelmed the available treatments.

In the early hours of the morning, the patient succumbed to the complications. The loss was profound, a stark reminder of the relentless nature of Factor XI deficiency. The patient's journey had been marked by a constant struggle against a condition that left no room for error.

Reflecting on the case, I was struck by the courage and tenacity the patient had shown throughout the years. The patient's life was a testament to the human spirit's ability to endure and adapt in the face of seemingly insurmountable challenges. The medical journey had been a learning experience, highlighting both the advancements and limitations of current treatments for rare bleeding disorders.

In the aftermath, I continued to follow the developments in gene therapy and other innovative treatments for hemophilia. The patient's story reinforced the importance of ongoing research and the need for more effective and accessible treatments for rare conditions. It also underscored the importance of empathy and support for patients navigating the complexities of chronic illness.

The patient's legacy lived on in the lessons learned and the ongoing quest for better treatments. Each new patient with a bleeding disorder reminded me of the delicate balance we must strive to achieve and the continuous pursuit of medical progress. The patient's story was a poignant chapter in my career, a reminder of the fragility of life and the resilience of the human spirit in the face of adversity.

Chapter 6
HALLERMANN-STREIFF SYNDROME

IT WAS a crisp autumn morning when I first encountered the patient who would profoundly impact my career. My medical practice was nestled in the small town of Arborville, a place where everyone knew each other and unusual medical cases were scarce. The patient came to me with a constellation of symptoms that painted a picture unlike any I had seen before.

The patient's parents brought them in, expressing their concern over developmental delays and a series of physical abnormalities. Upon first glance, it was clear that this was not a typical case. The patient's face was marked by a distinctive, almost bird-like appearance, with a beaked nose and underdeveloped jaw. Their head was disproportionately large compared to their body, and their skin was thin and delicate, almost translucent in places. These features, combined with sparse hair and dental issues, pointed me toward a rare diagnosis.

I meticulously conducted a series of physical examinations, took detailed family histories, and ordered a battery of tests. The patient exhibited dwarfism, with short stature evident even at their young age. The eyes were a particular concern; they were unusually large and bulging, suggesting potential ocular complications. Despite their fragile appearance, the patient was alert and inquisitive, a testament to the human spirit's indomitable strength.

As the results trickled in, the pieces of the puzzle began to fit together. The combination of craniofacial anomalies, dental issues, and growth deficiencies led me to suspect Hallermann-Streiff Syndrome, a rare genetic disorder. A referral to a geneticist confirmed my suspicions. Hallermann-Streiff Syndrome, characterized by such distinct and severe symptoms, was a daunting diagnosis for any family to receive.

Breaking the news to the patient's family was one of the hardest moments of my career. I explained the condition's genetic basis, detailing how it typically arises from new mutations rather than being inherited from the parents. I outlined the prognosis and the myriad challenges the patient would face throughout their life.

The parents listened intently, their faces a mixture of fear, sadness, and a determination that belied their external calm.

The treatment plan was multifaceted, addressing both immediate and long-term needs. Regular visits to a variety of specialists were essential. An ophthalmologist monitored the patient closely for signs of cataracts, glaucoma, and other potential eye issues. Given the patient's fragile bones, a pediatric orthopedist was involved to address skeletal abnormalities and manage any fractures that might occur.

Dental care was another critical component of the treatment plan. The patient had hypodontia, a condition where some teeth are missing, and the existing teeth were often malformed. Regular visits to a pediatric dentist helped manage these issues, and we explored the possibility of orthodontic interventions to improve function and appearance as the patient grew older.

One of the most significant challenges was addressing the patient's respiratory difficulties. The underdeveloped nasal passages and small mouth made breathing a constant struggle, especially during sleep. A sleep study revealed severe obstructive sleep apnea, necessitating the use of a CPAP machine to ensure the patient could breathe properly at night. Additionally, consultations with an ENT specialist led to discussions about potential surgical interventions to alleviate some of these issues.

Despite the best efforts of our multidisciplinary team, the patient faced daily challenges. Their growth was stunted, and their physical appearance led to social difficulties. The parents were dedicated advocates, ensuring their child received the best care and support possible. They worked closely with teachers and school administrators to create a supportive educational environment that accommodated the patient's needs.

As the patient grew older, new challenges emerged. Adolescence is a difficult time for any child, but for the patient, it was particularly harsh. The physical differences became more pronounced, and the social isolation more acute. We arranged for counseling and support groups to help the patient navigate these tumultuous years. The patient's spirit, though tested, remained remarkably steadfast.

Throughout this time, regular medical check-ups and treatments continued. The patient underwent multiple surgeries to correct skeletal deformities and address respiratory issues. Each procedure carried its risks, but the potential benefits outweighed them. The patient's family was always present, their unwavering support a beacon of hope.

Despite our best efforts, the patient's condition began to deteriorate in their late teens. The frequent respiratory infections became harder to manage, and their overall health declined. The delicate balance we had maintained for years was tipping.

In the final months, the patient was in and out of the hospital. Pneumonia became a recurrent issue, and their frail body struggled to fight off infections. The medical team did everything possible to provide comfort and manage symptoms, but it was clear that we were nearing the end of our battle.

I will never forget the day when the patient's parents made the heart-wrenching decision to transition to palliative care. They wanted their child to be at home, surrounded by loved ones, rather than in a sterile hospital environment. We arranged for home hospice care, ensuring that all necessary medical support was in place to keep the patient comfortable.

During those final weeks, I visited the patient frequently. Each visit was a reminder of the fragility of life and the incredible strength of the human spirit. The patient's family created a peaceful and loving environment, filled with music, laughter, and memories. The patient, despite their condition, maintained a quiet grace and composure.

The end came one peaceful evening. Surrounded

by family, the patient slipped away quietly. The parents called me immediately, and I arrived shortly after to confirm the passing. It was a moment of profound sadness but also one of relief, knowing that the patient was no longer in pain.

In the days that followed, I reflected on the journey we had all undertaken. Hallermann-Streiff Syndrome is a rare and relentless condition, but the patient and their family faced it with a strength and tenacity that was truly remarkable. Their journey was marked by challenges and heartaches, but also by love, perseverance, and moments of joy.

The patient's legacy lives on in my practice. Their case has taught me the importance of compassion, the necessity of a multidisciplinary approach, and the profound impact of family support in managing chronic conditions. I have shared their story with medical students and colleagues, emphasizing the importance of holistic care and the need to see beyond the disease to the person living with it.

In the end, while the patient's life was brief and fraught with difficulties, it was also a testament to the enduring power of the human spirit. Their courage and the dedication of their family serve as a powerful reminder of what it means to live with grace in the face of adversity.

Chapter 7
JANSEN TYPE METAPHYSEAL CHONDRODYSPLASIA

I REMEMBER the day the patient walked into my clinic, a small, timid figure whose gait was noticeably irregular. The patient was a child, no more than ten years old, accompanied by a worried parent. The air in the room seemed thick with concern, and I could sense the heavy burden of fear that hung over them. Little did I know that this would mark the beginning of a long and arduous journey through a rare and challenging medical condition.

The patient's symptoms had started with a slight limp that progressively worsened over several months. There were complaints of persistent pain in the legs and difficulty in performing everyday activities. These signs, combined with the noticeable bowing of the legs, raised my suspicions of a skeletal disorder. After a thorough physical examination, I ordered a series of X-rays to get a clearer picture of what was happening internally.

The X-ray results were revealing. They showed irregularities in the metaphyses of the long bones, a characteristic flaring that suggested an abnormality in bone development. Additionally, there were signs of metaphyseal dysplasia—irregular, splayed, and widened metaphyseal regions that indicated a disruption in normal bone growth. With these findings, I decided to proceed with more specialized imaging, including a CT scan, to further assess the extent of the bone deformities.

As I awaited the imaging results, I delved into the patient's medical history. There were no significant illnesses or injuries that could account for the current condition. The family history, however, revealed a potential clue: a distant relative had been diagnosed with a rare genetic disorder affecting bone develop-ment. This piece of information, combined with the imaging results, pointed me towards a diagnosis that, though rare, fit the clinical picture—Jansen Type Meta-physeal Chondrodysplasia (JMC).

JMC is a rare skeletal disorder caused by mutations in the PTH1R gene, which encodes the receptor for parathyroid hormone and parathyroid hormone-related peptide. These mutations lead to abnormal signaling pathways that disrupt normal bone growth and development. With the diagnosis in mind, I explained to the patient's family the nature of the condition, its genetic basis, and the implications for the patient's health.

Given the rarity of JMC, the treatment options were limited and primarily focused on managing symptoms and improving the patient's quality of life. The first step was to address the pain and improve mobility. I prescribed a regimen of pain management medications, including nonsteroidal anti-inflammatory drugs (NSAIDs) and, when necessary, more potent analgesics. Physical therapy was also essential to strengthen the muscles around the affected joints, improve flexibility, and reduce the risk of further deformities.

Regular follow-up visits were scheduled to monitor the patient's progress and adjust the treatment plan as needed. During these visits, we tracked the patient's growth and development, looking for any signs of worsening or new symptoms. Despite our best efforts, the patient continued to experience significant pain and mobility issues, necessitating further intervention.

As the patient grew older, the skeletal deformities became more pronounced, and the pain more severe. The limited options for curative treatment forced us to consider surgical interventions to correct some of the more debilitating deformities. The decision to proceed with surgery was not taken lightly. We consulted with orthopedic specialists who had experience with similar cases, and together we formulated a surgical plan aimed at correcting the most critical deformities and improving the patient's overall function.

The first surgery involved osteotomies to correct the bowing of the legs. The procedure was intricate and required precise planning and execution. The orthopedic surgeon made careful cuts in the bones to realign them and used internal fixation devices to hold the bones in the correct position as they healed. The surgery was followed by a lengthy recovery period, during which the patient remained under close observation to monitor for complications such as infections or issues with bone healing.

Post-operative care included intensive physical therapy to aid in the rehabilitation process. The patient's determination and the support of their family were evident during this challenging time. The exercises were often painful, and progress was slow, but the goal of improved mobility and reduced pain provided a glimmer of hope.

Despite the successful surgical interventions, the underlying genetic disorder continued to present challenges. The patient faced recurrent episodes of pain and required ongoing medical management. We explored various medications and treatments to manage the chronic pain, including bisphosphonates to strengthen the bones and reduce the risk of fractures.

Over the years, the patient's condition remained a delicate balance between managing symptoms and maintaining as normal a life as possible. There were periods of relative stability interspersed with flare-ups of pain and difficulty. Each setback was met with adjustments in treatment and a renewed effort to provide the best possible care.

As the patient transitioned into adolescence, the physical and emotional challenges became more pronounced. The visible skeletal deformities and limited mobility affected the patient's self-esteem and social interactions. Counseling and psychological support were integrated into the treatment plan to address these aspects and provide a holistic approach to care.

Throughout this journey, the patient demonstrated an incredible fortitude. Each visit to the clinic was a reminder of the resilience that lies within the human spirit, even in the face of such a daunting condition. The family's unwavering support played a crucial role in navigating the complexities of JMC, and their dedication to the patient's well-being was truly inspiring.

In the latter years of the patient's care, we explored emerging treatments and participated in clinical trials aimed at finding more effective therapies for JMC. These trials offered a ray of hope, but the rarity of the condition meant that progress was slow and often fraught with uncertainty.

The patient's condition, while managed as best as possible, remained a constant presence. There were times when the pain and limitations felt overwhelming, but the patient and their family continued to approach each day with a sense of determination. The medical team worked tirelessly to provide the best possible care, continually adapting to the evolving needs of the patient.

Ultimately, the patient's journey with JMC was one of both struggle and perseverance. The medical challenges were immense, and the road to managing the condition was long and often arduous. Yet, through it all, there was an unwavering commitment to improving the patient's quality of life and providing the support needed to navigate the complexities of this rare disorder.

Reflecting on the patient's story, I am reminded of the profound impact that rare diseases have on individuals and their families. The journey is often filled with uncertainty and difficulty, but it is also marked by moments of triumph and the strength of the human spirit. The experience underscored the importance of continued research and advancements in medical science to provide better outcomes for those affected by rare conditions like JMC.

In the end, the patient's story is a testament to the enduring power of hope and the relentless pursuit of a better life, even in the face of formidable odds. It serves as a reminder that, as medical professionals, our role extends beyond treatment to being a source of support and encouragement for those who rely on us in their most vulnerable moments.

Chapter 8
MAY HEGGLIN ANOMALY

I HAD BEEN PRACTICING medicine for over two decades when the case of May-Hegglin Anomaly crossed my path. It was a routine day in the clinic, and I was working through a stack of patient files when I first encountered the patient. Their initial presentation was not alarming: they had come in for a routine check-up, a bit more fatigued than usual, and with occasional episodes of unexplained bruising.

During the examination, I noticed petechiae—small, red spots on the skin indicative of minor hemorrhages. The patient also had a few larger, purplish bruises that stood out starkly against their skin. These findings were peculiar, and my mind immediately raced through possible causes: clotting disorders, platelet abnormalities, or even some form of vasculitis.

Blood work was the obvious next step. I ordered a complete blood count (CBC) with a differential and a peripheral blood smear. The CBC revealed thrombocytopenia, a lower than normal platelet count. This finding corroborated the physical signs and hinted at a possible hematological disorder. The peripheral blood smear, however, revealed the defining clue: large platelets, almost the size of red blood cells, and the presence of Döhle-like bodies—bluish-gray inclusions within the white blood cells.

These findings pointed towards a rare genetic disorder: May-Hegglin Anomaly (MHA). This condition, characterized by thrombocytopenia, giant platelets, and Döhle-like bodies in granulocytes, is a type of MYH9-related disorder. MYH9 gene mutations are responsible for these abnormalities. With these results in hand, I explained the situation to the patient and scheduled further tests, including genetic testing, to confirm the diagnosis.

The genetic test results took a few weeks, during which the patient's symptoms remained relatively stable. When the results finally arrived, they confirmed my suspicion: a mutation in the MYH9 gene. This confirmation allowed me to provide a definitive diagnosis of May-Hegglin Anomaly.

The patient's immediate reaction was a mix of

relief and confusion. On one hand, they were relieved to have a name for their symptoms; on the other, the rarity of the condition and the genetic implications were daunting. I spent considerable time explaining the nature of the disorder, its hereditary aspects, and potential complications.

Management of May-Hegglin Anomaly is primarily symptomatic. The patient's thrombocytopenia put them at risk of bleeding, particularly in cases of trauma or surgery. I advised the patient to avoid activities that could result in injury and to be vigilant for signs of bleeding.

Over the following months, the patient adhered to the recommendations diligently. However, despite these precautions, they experienced episodes of spontaneous bleeding, such as nosebleeds and gastrointestinal bleeding, which required hospitalization and transfusions of platelets and red blood cells. Each incident was a stark reminder of the fragility of their condition.

The treatment protocol involved regular monitoring of platelet counts and bleeding parameters. Given the patient's recurrent bleeding episodes, I initiated treatment with antifibrinolytic agents to reduce the risk of bleeding. Additionally, I collaborated with a hematologist to explore further options. We discussed the potential use of thrombopoietin receptor agonists, which could stimulate platelet production, but decided against it due to the associated risks and limited evidence of efficacy in MHA.

During one of the follow-up visits, the patient mentioned experiencing visual disturbances. Concerned about a possible complication, I referred them to an ophthalmologist. The ophthalmological examination revealed the presence of cataracts, another known association with MYH9-related disorders. This necessitated further intervention to prevent deterioration of vision. The patient underwent cataract surgery, which, fortunately, was successful and uneventful.

As time went on, the patient became a regular at the clinic. We developed a routine of frequent checkups, laboratory tests, and consultations with various specialists. The patient's determination was remarkable; they adapted their lifestyle to manage their condition, always maintaining a positive outlook despite the challenges.

However, the chronic nature of the disorder began to take its toll. The patient's quality of life was significantly impacted by the constant vigilance required to manage their symptoms. They became increasingly fatigued and occasionally expressed feelings of frustration and helplessness. It was during these times that I focused on providing emotional support and reassurance, emphasizing the importance of a multidisciplinary approach in managing their condition.

Despite all efforts, there came a time when the patient's condition began to deteriorate more rapidly. They developed severe gastrointestinal bleeding that was unresponsive to conventional treatments. This led to multiple hospital admissions and a significant decline in their overall health. The once bright and hopeful demeanor was now overshadowed by the weariness of constant battles with their own body.

During one particularly severe episode, the patient was admitted to the intensive care unit. The bleeding was relentless, and despite aggressive transfusions and medical interventions, their condition worsened. The multidisciplinary team, including hematologists, gastroenterologists, and critical care specialists, worked tirelessly to stabilize the patient. However, the severity of the bleeding and the underlying platelet dysfunction posed insurmountable challenges.

The patient's family was informed of the critical nature of the situation. It was a heartbreaking moment for everyone involved. Despite all the advanced medical interventions, the patient's condition continued to decline. The body, worn out by constant bleeding and the strain of numerous medical procedures, finally succumbed.

The patient passed away in the early hours of a quiet morning. The sense of loss was profound. I spent some time reflecting on their journey, the courage they had shown, and the relentless fight they had put up against a rare and unforgiving disorder.

In the aftermath, I reached out to the patient's family, offering my condolences and support. The experience left a lasting impact on me as a physician. It reinforced the importance of compassion, continuous learning, and the need to support patients and their families through the highs and lows of chronic illness management.

May-Hegglin Anomaly had proven to be a formidable adversary. It highlighted the limitations of current medical knowledge and the importance of ongoing research to better understand and manage rare genetic disorders. The patient's journey was a stark reminder of the fragility of life and the strength of the human spirit in facing such adversities.

In the end, while the patient did not survive, their battle with May-Hegglin Anomaly underscored the need for a holistic approach to patient care, one that integrates medical treatment with emotional and psychological support. It was a poignant reminder that, as physicians, our role extends beyond curing diseases to alleviating suffering and providing comfort in the face of life's inevitable challenges.

The case of May-Hegglin Anomaly taught me more than I had ever learned from textbooks or lectures. It was a journey through the complexities of human health and the uncharted territories of rare genetic disorders. Though the patient's life was cut short, their legacy lives on in the lessons learned and the relentless pursuit of knowledge and better care for those who follow.

Chapter 9
OTOPALATODIGITAL SYNDROME TYPE I

I FIRST ENCOUNTERED the patient on a dreary autumn morning. The weather seemed to mirror the atmosphere within the walls of our hospital—grey, cold, and heavy with uncertainty. As a seasoned physician, I had faced numerous medical challenges, yet the intricacies of rare genetic disorders never ceased to intrigue me. The patient, a young individual, had been referred to our facility after a series of perplexing symptoms and inconclusive diagnoses from other hospitals.

Upon reviewing the patient's medical records, a pattern began to emerge. The patient had a history of skeletal abnormalities, most notably in the facial structure and digits. The midface appeared underdeveloped, with a flattened nasal bridge and widely spaced eyes.

The fingers were short and broad, reminiscent of a condition I had only read about in medical journals. My initial suspicion was a rare genetic disorder, but the exact nature eluded me until further tests could be conducted.

The patient had been living with these abnormalities for years, enduring not only physical discomfort but also the psychological burden of being different. Social interactions were fraught with challenges, and the patient had faced considerable adversity due to their appearance. It was evident that the psychological scars were as deep as the physical ones.

Our first course of action was to perform a thorough physical examination and order a series of imaging studies. The radiographs revealed significant skeletal dysplasia. The bones of the skull, particularly the frontal and parietal bones, showed signs of early fusion, a condition known as craniosynostosis. This abnormal fusion leads to an altered shape of the head and can potentially impact brain development if not addressed. The hands and feet exhibited characteristic features: short, broad digits with abnormal spacing between them. These findings were suggestive of a rare disorder known as Otopalatodigital Syndrome Type I (OPD I).

Otopalatodigital Syndrome Type I is a genetic

disorder caused by mutations in the FLNA gene, which encodes for the protein filamin A. This protein plays a crucial role in the development of the cytoskeleton, the structure that helps cells maintain their shape and internal organization. Mutations in this gene disrupt normal skeletal development, leading to the characteristic features observed in the patient.

With a probable diagnosis in hand, I proceeded to explain the condition to the patient and their family. The complexity of genetic disorders can be overwhelming, and I aimed to provide a clear understanding of what lay ahead. The condition, though not curable, could be managed to improve quality of life. Our treatment plan focused on addressing the most pressing issues: craniosynostosis and skeletal deformities.

Surgery was the cornerstone of our treatment approach. The patient underwent cranial vault remodeling to correct the premature fusion of the skull bones. This procedure was intricate, requiring collaboration with a skilled team of neurosurgeons and craniofacial surgeons. The goal was to create more space for the growing brain and improve the overall shape of the head. The surgery was successful, albeit not without its risks. Post-operative care involved meticulous monitoring to prevent complications such as infection or increased intracranial pressure.

While the cranial surgery addressed the immediate threat to the patient's neurological development, the skeletal abnormalities in the limbs required a different approach. Orthopedic interventions, including corrective surgeries on the hands and feet, were planned in stages. The first surgery aimed to realign the bones in the hands to improve functionality and dexterity. This was followed by procedures on the feet to address the abnormal spacing and enhance mobility. Each surgery was a step towards a better quality of life, though the journey was long and fraught with challenges.

Throughout this period, the patient's spirit and fortitude were remarkable. The recovery process was arduous, involving extensive physiotherapy and rehabilitation. Each small victory, whether it was the ability to grasp objects more effectively or walk with greater ease, was a testament to the patient's indomitable will. The psychological support provided by our team of counselors and therapists was invaluable, helping the patient navigate the emotional and mental hurdles that accompanied their physical recovery.

Genetic counseling was another critical component of our treatment plan. Understanding the hereditary nature of OPD I was essential for the patient and their family. We discussed the implications of the disorder, the risks of passing it on to future generations, and the options available for family planning. Knowledge, we believed, was empowering, and our aim was to equip the patient and their family with as much information as possible to make informed decisions about their future.

As months turned into years, the patient's condition stabilized. The surgeries had significantly improved their physical capabilities, and the intensive rehabilitation had borne fruit. The patient's hands, though still showing signs of the disorder, were far more functional than before. Walking, once a laborious task, had become more manageable. Socially, the patient began to reintegrate, finding solace in new friendships and activities that celebrated their unique strengths.

However, OPD I is a lifelong condition, and vigilance was necessary. Regular follow-ups became part of our routine, ensuring that any new complications were promptly addressed. The patient's growth and development were closely monitored, with periodic imaging studies and physical examinations. The team remained proactive, ready to intervene should any new issues arise.

One of the significant concerns with OPD I is the potential for hearing loss, as the disorder can affect the structures of the inner ear. We conducted regular audiological assessments to monitor the patient's hearing.

When a mild hearing impairment was detected, we promptly fitted the patient with hearing aids. This intervention, though minor in the grand scheme of things, had a profound impact on the patient's ability to communicate and engage with the world around them.

Over time, the patient's story became one of adaptation and perseverance. While OPD I had imposed numerous limitations, it had also shaped a character marked by tenacity and determination. The patient's journey was a testament to the human spirit's capacity to endure and thrive despite overwhelming odds.

Reflecting on this case, I was reminded of the profound impact that rare genetic disorders can have on individuals and their families. The medical journey is not just about treating symptoms but about understanding the person behind the condition. It is about acknowledging their struggles, celebrating their victories, and supporting them through every challenge.

The patient's journey was not one of complete healing, for OPD I is a condition that cannot be cured. Yet, it was a journey of significant improvement, both physically and emotionally. The surgeries and therapies had transformed the patient's life, enabling them to achieve a level of functionality that had once seemed unattainable. The psychological support had fortified their mental resilience, helping them navigate the complexities of living with a chronic condition.

As a physician, cases like this one are a stark reminder of the importance of a holistic approach to healthcare. It is not enough to treat the physical manifestations of a disease; one must also address the emotional and psychological dimensions. The patient's journey was a collaborative effort, involving surgeons, therapists, genetic counselors, and, most importantly, the patient and their family. Each played a crucial role in the tapestry of care that was woven around the patient.

The autumn morning when I first met the patient now seemed a distant memory, overshadowed by the progress and transformations that had since unfolded. The journey through shadows had led to a place of light and hope, a place where the patient could envision a future not defined by their condition but by their capabilities and dreams.

In the end, the patient's story was one of remarkable perseverance. It highlighted the incredible advances in medical science that can offer hope and improvement to those with rare genetic disorders. It also underscored the unyielding human spirit's ability to adapt, endure, and flourish despite the most daunting challenges. The patient's journey was a powerful reminder that while we may not always be able to cure, we can always strive to heal, support, and uplift those in our care.

As I watched the patient walk out of the hospital on a crisp spring morning, their steps steady and confident, I felt a profound sense of fulfillment. The journey was far from over, but the strides we had made together were monumental. It was a journey marked by struggle and triumph, a journey that reaffirmed my commitment to the practice of medicine and the care of those who place their trust in our hands.

Chapter 10
RELAPSING POLYCHONDRITIS

I FIRST ENCOUNTERED the patient on an unusually hot day in June, the kind of day that made even the sterile halls of the hospital feel oppressive. They came in complaining of what they initially described as "strange, recurrent bouts of pain and swelling" in various parts of their body. As a seasoned physician, I had seen my fair share of puzzling cases, but the patient's symptoms were particularly perplexing.

The patient's ears were swollen and red, as if they had been severely sunburned. Their nose was tender to the touch, and they reported pain in their joints that seemed to migrate from one location to another. The symptoms were reminiscent of an inflammatory condition, but the specifics did not align neatly with any single diagnosis I could readily think of.

I began with a thorough examination and a battery of tests. Blood tests showed elevated levels of inflammatory markers, and imaging revealed inflammation in the cartilage of the patient's ears and nose. There was no evidence of infection, and the usual autoimmune suspects such as lupus and rheumatoid arthritis were ruled out. The patient's medical history was unremarkable, with no prior indications of autoimmune disorders. This left me with a challenging diagnostic puzzle.

After consulting with colleagues and reviewing the literature, I began to suspect Relapsing Polychondritis (RP), a rare autoimmune condition characterized by recurrent inflammation of cartilaginous tissues. The patient's symptoms matched the classic presentation of RP: recurrent episodes of painful, swollen cartilage in the ears, nose, and joints. Though rare, this diagnosis made sense given the patient's presentation.

Confirming the diagnosis of RP required more than just clinical suspicion. I ordered a biopsy of the cartilage in the patient's ear, which revealed the hallmark features of RP: inflammation and degradation of the cartilage. The diagnosis was confirmed, and I sat down to devise a treatment plan.

Relapsing Polychondritis is a chronic condition, often requiring lifelong management. The primary goal is to reduce inflammation and prevent further damage to the cartilage. The first line of treatment involved corticosteroids to control the acute flare-ups. I prescribed a high dose of prednisone to start, with a plan to taper down as the inflammation came under control. The patient was also started on a course of nonsteroidal anti-inflammatory drugs (NSAIDs) to help manage pain and inflammation.

In addition to medication, I emphasized the importance of monitoring for potential complications. RP can affect other systems, including the respiratory tract, heart, and eyes, leading to life-threatening complications. Regular follow-up appointments were scheduled to keep a close watch on the patient's progress and any new symptoms that might arise.

Initially, the treatment seemed effective. The patient reported a significant reduction in pain and swelling, and their quality of life improved. However, as with many autoimmune conditions, the road to management was far from smooth. Within a few months, the patient began to experience flare-ups despite the medication. The symptoms were unpredictable and debilitating, often flaring up without warning and causing significant distress.

Given the recurrent nature of the patient's symptoms, I decided to introduce additional immunosuppressive therapy. Methotrexate, a disease-modifying antirheumatic drug (DMARD), was added to the treatment regimen. This medication works by dampening the immune system's activity, thereby reducing inflammation. The goal was to achieve better control of the disease and reduce the reliance on corticosteroids, which can have significant long-term side effects.

Managing the side effects of the medication became a crucial aspect of the patient's care. Corticosteroids, while effective, come with a host of potential complications, including weight gain, hypertension, osteoporosis, and increased risk of infections. The patient was counseled on these risks and monitored closely. Bone density scans were conducted to keep an eye on potential osteoporosis, and the patient was prescribed calcium and vitamin D supplements as a preventive measure.

Despite the challenges, the patient demonstrated a remarkable capacity to adapt to their circumstances. They adhered to the treatment plan diligently, attended all follow-up appointments, and communicated openly about their symptoms and any side effects they experienced. This proactive approach played a crucial role in managing the disease effectively.

Over time, the flare-ups became less frequent and less severe. The combination of corticosteroids and methotrexate seemed to stabilize the patient's condition. While there were still occasional setbacks, the overall trend was positive. The patient's quality of life improved, and they were able to resume many of their normal activities.

However, the unpredictable nature of RP meant that vigilance was always necessary. One of the most concerning aspects of RP is its potential to affect the respiratory tract. Inflammation of the trachea and bronchi can lead to airway obstruction, a potentially life-threatening complication. To monitor for this, regular pulmonary function tests were conducted. Fortunately, the patient did not show any signs of respiratory involvement, but this remained a key focus of their ongoing care.

As months turned into years, the patient's condition remained relatively stable. They experienced occasional flare-ups, but these were managed effectively with adjustments to their medication regimen. The long-term use of immunosuppressive therapy required regular monitoring of blood counts and liver function, but the patient tolerated the treatment well overall.

Despite the chronic nature of RP, the patient managed to maintain a positive outlook. They adapted to their new normal, finding ways to manage the disease while still enjoying life. Their determination was inspiring and a testament to the human spirit's capacity to endure and adapt in the face of adversity.

However, RP is a relentless foe, and despite our best efforts, it can still pose serious threats. Several years into the patient's journey, they developed a new, concerning symptom: hoarseness and difficulty breathing. These symptoms suggested potential involvement of the respiratory tract, a dreaded complication of RP. An urgent bronchoscopy was performed, revealing inflammation and narrowing of the trachea.

This complication necessitated a more aggressive treatment approach. High-dose intravenous corticosteroids were administered to quickly reduce the inflammation, and the patient was hospitalized for close monitoring. The goal was to prevent the airway from becoming critically obstructed while controlling the inflammation. The patient responded well to the treatment, and the airway obstruction was relieved. However, this episode highlighted the constant vigilance required in managing RP and the ever-present risk of serious complications.

The patient was discharged with a revised treatment plan, including a higher maintenance dose of corticosteroids and an additional immunosuppressant, azathioprine, to better control the disease. Regular follow-ups with a pulmonologist were also arranged to monitor the respiratory tract more closely.

Despite this setback, the patient continued to demonstrate an impressive capacity to adapt and endure. They adjusted to the new treatment regimen and remained proactive in their care. The support of their family and friends played a crucial role in helping them navigate the challenges of living with a chronic, unpredictable disease.

As time passed, the patient's condition stabilized once again. They continued to experience occasional flare-ups, but these were managed effectively with the adjusted treatment plan. The patient remained vigilant, attending all follow-up appointments and promptly reporting any new symptoms.

Reflecting on the patient's journey, I was struck by the complexity and unpredictability of Relapsing Poly-chondritis. It is a disease that demands constant vigilance and adaptability, both from the patient and the healthcare team. The patient's story is a testament to the importance of a comprehensive, multidisciplinary approach to managing chronic diseases, as well as the critical role of patient education and support.

In the end, the patient's journey with Relapsing Polychondritis was one of ongoing management rather than a definitive cure. While there were significant challenges and setbacks, the patient's proactive approach to their care and their capacity to adapt made a crucial difference in their quality of life. They continued to live with RP, but it did not define them. Instead, it became one aspect of their life, one that they managed with courage and determination.

Their story is a reminder of the importance of resilience in the face of chronic illness, not only for the patients who live with these conditions but also for the healthcare professionals who support them. Each day presents new challenges and opportunities, and it is through perseverance and adaptability that we find the strength to overcome them.

As a physician, I learned a great deal from the patient's journey. Their case reinforced the importance of listening to patients, understanding their experiences, and working collaboratively to develop and adjust treatment plans. It also underscored the need for ongoing research and education to better understand and manage complex autoimmune diseases like Relapsing Polychondritis.

In the end, while the patient's journey with RP was marked by many challenges, it was also a story of hope and perseverance. Through effective management, supportive care, and a proactive approach, the patient was able to navigate the ups and downs of their condition, finding ways to live a fulfilling life despite the challenges posed by Relapsing Polychondritis.

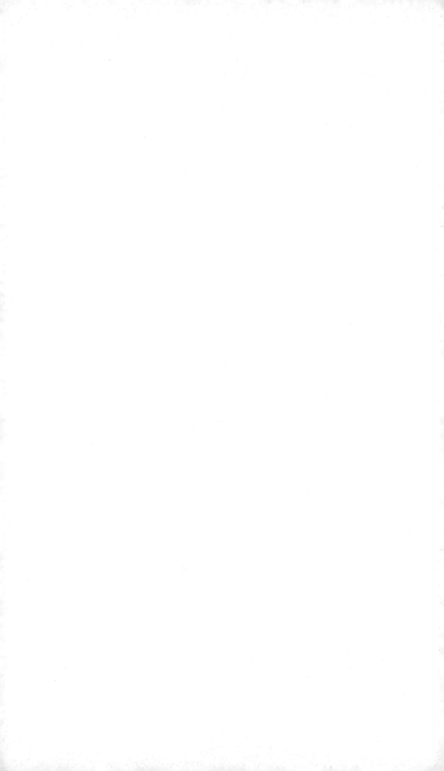

Chapter 11
PACHYONYCHIA CONGENITA

THE PATIENT CAME into my office on a brisk autumn morning, their footsteps tentative and careful. The usual bright energy of the season outside my window stood in stark contrast to the subdued atmosphere inside my examination room. As a dermatologist with years of experience, I had seen numerous cases of various skin conditions, but the patient's presentation was unique. They were young, in their early thirties, and appeared otherwise healthy, but their hands and feet told a different story.

Thickened, discolored nails adorned their fingers and toes, curling inwards and creating a grotesque landscape of keratin. The patient recounted a history of painful blisters and calluses on the soles of their feet and palms, exacerbated by even minimal physical activity. Their voice, though calm, carried the weight of long-standing discomfort and frustration.

I began my examination with a thorough inspection of the nails. Pachyonychia Congenita (PC) crossed my mind almost immediately. This rare genetic disorder, characterized by nail dystrophy, painful plantar keratoderma, and oral leukokeratosis, seemed to fit the symptoms perfectly. Still, differential diagnosis was necessary. Conditions such as fungal infections, psoriasis, and lichen planus needed to be ruled out.

I ordered a series of tests. A nail clipping was sent for histopathological examination and a genetic test was arranged to confirm the presence of mutations in the keratin genes KRT6A, KRT6B, KRT16, or KRT17. In the meantime, I prescribed a topical urea cream to alleviate some of the thickening and pain, knowing it was a temporary measure at best.

The histopathology came back first, showing hyperkeratosis and acanthosis without signs of fungal infection. The genetic test took longer, but when the results arrived, they confirmed my suspicions. The patient had a mutation in the KRT16 gene, solidifying the diagnosis of Pachyonychia Congenita.

I explained the genetic nature of the disease to the patient, detailing how the mutation affected the keratin production, leading to the thickened nails and painful calluses. There was no cure, but there were treatment options to manage the symptoms and improve the quality of life. The patient listened intently, their expression a mix of relief at having a diagnosis and apprehension about the chronic nature of the condition.

We embarked on a treatment plan focusing on symptom management. Pain relief was paramount. I prescribed oral analgesics and recommended warm foot soaks to soften the calluses. Keratolytic agents like salicylic acid and lactic acid were applied to reduce the hyperkeratosis. The patient was advised to wear comfortable, cushioned footwear to minimize pressure on their feet.

Regular follow-ups were scheduled to monitor the progression and efficacy of the treatments. Over the next few months, the patient adhered to the regimen diligently. There were some improvements; the calluses became more manageable, and the pain less intense. However, new blisters would occasionally form, reminding us of the relentless nature of the disorder.

I also suggested the patient join a support group for individuals with PC. Sharing experiences with others who faced similar challenges could provide emotional support and practical advice. The patient found solace in these interactions, gaining valuable tips on managing their condition.

Despite our efforts, there were days when the patient's condition worsened. The winter months were particularly harsh. The cold weather aggravated their symptoms, making walking excruciatingly painful. On such days, the patient would often stay indoors, using the time to rest and recover.

One spring, a promising clinical trial for a novel topical siRNA treatment targeting the mutant keratin gene was announced. This treatment aimed to silence the defective gene and potentially reduce the symptoms. After discussing the potential risks and benefits, the patient decided to participate in the trial.

The treatment required bi-weekly applications of the siRNA cream, and the patient reported back to the clinic regularly for monitoring. The initial results were encouraging. The thickness of the nails began to decrease, and the frequency of new blisters reduced. It seemed as though we were on the cusp of a breakthrough.

However, about six months into the trial, the patient developed a severe skin infection at one of the application sites. The infection was aggressive, rapidly spreading and causing significant discomfort. The patient was immediately withdrawn from the trial and started on a course of potent antibiotics. The infection eventually subsided, but it left behind scarring and a renewed sense of caution.

This setback was disheartening, but it did not deter us. The patient resumed the previous treatment regimen, and we explored other avenues, including genetic counseling and new emerging therapies. Throughout these trials, the patient demonstrated a remarkable ability to adapt and maintain a hopeful outlook despite the chronic nature of their condition.

Several years passed, marked by incremental improvements and occasional setbacks. The patient's condition remained stable, though not cured. The pain was more manageable, and the nails, while still thickened, were less so than before. We continued to monitor and adjust the treatment plan as new research and therapies emerged.

Eventually, the patient's health began to decline due to unrelated causes. The constant pain and difficulty in walking had taken a toll on their overall physical health, leading to complications such as muscle atrophy and joint issues. Despite these challenges, the patient continued to engage with the support group, drawing strength and inspiration from the shared experiences.

In the final months, the patient's condition deteriorated rapidly. The underlying genetic disorder, compounded by age and other health issues, proved too much for their body to withstand. Surrounded by family and friends, the patient passed away peacefully.

Reflecting on the patient's journey, I felt a deep sense of respect and admiration for their fortitude. Pachyonychia Congenita had imposed numerous challenges, but the patient faced them with an unwavering spirit. Their experience underscored the importance of patient-centered care, the need for continued research, and the value of emotional support in managing chronic conditions.

In the end, while we had not achieved a cure, we had made strides in improving the quality of life for the patient. Their journey contributed to a better understanding of Pachyonychia Congenita and paved the way for future advancements in treatment. The patient's legacy lived on in the ongoing research and the support community they had helped to build, offering hope to others facing similar challenges.

Chapter 12
NECROTIZING ENTEROCOLITIS

IN THE QUIET hours of the night, the hospital had a different rhythm. The corridors were dimly lit, the usual bustle of daytime activities reduced to a muted hum. It was during these hours that I often found myself reflecting on the fragility of life and the delicate balance we, as doctors, strive to maintain. One such night, I encountered a case that would forever etch itself into my memory—the patient with Necrotizing Enterocolitis (NEC).

The patient was a premature infant, born at just 28 weeks. The neonatal intensive care unit (NICU) had become their fragile sanctuary, a place where every breath was a victory and every heartbeat a triumph. The baby had been in our care for two weeks, their tiny form connected to an array of monitors and machines that beeped and whirred in a constant symphony of vigilance.

It was on a Tuesday morning when the first signs of trouble emerged. The patient's abdomen appeared distended, and there was a noticeable discoloration—a bluish hue that set off alarms in my mind. The infant's feeding tolerance had decreased, and there was an alarming increase in gastric residuals. These symptoms, though subtle, hinted at a more sinister undercurrent. A blood sample was drawn, revealing a concerning shift in white blood cell counts and a rise in inflammatory markers.

I suspected NEC, a severe gastrointestinal disease primarily affecting premature infants. It involves the death of tissue in the intestines, leading to inflammation and, potentially, a perforation of the intestinal wall. The exact cause remains elusive, but contributing factors include the immaturity of the infant's intestines, bacterial infection, and compromised blood flow.

The patient's condition deteriorated rapidly. Their belly became more distended, and the discoloration deepened. Radiographic imaging was ordered, revealing pneumatosis intestinalis—air within the intestinal wall—confirming the diagnosis of NEC. The sight of those dark, gas-filled loops of bowel on the X-ray filled me with a profound sense of urgency and dread.

Immediate intervention was crucial. The patient was placed on nothing by mouth (NPO) status to rest the intestines, and intravenous fluids were administered to maintain hydration and electrolyte balance. Broad-spectrum antibiotics were started to combat any bacterial infection. The delicate dance of medical management had begun, with the infant's life hanging by a thread.

The NICU team worked with an intensity born of experience and a deep-seated desire to save the smallest and most vulnerable among us. Parenteral nutrition was initiated to provide essential nutrients without burdening the compromised gut. We monitored the baby's vital signs with unwavering attention, every fluctuation in heart rate or blood pressure analyzed with painstaking care.

Despite our efforts, the patient's condition remained precarious. The distention worsened, and the baby's overall appearance grew more lethargic. Blood gases indicated metabolic acidosis, a sign that the body was struggling to maintain its delicate equilibrium. The decision to proceed with surgical intervention loomed ever closer—a daunting prospect given the patient's fragility.

Surgery was the last resort, a measure taken when all other interventions fail to halt the progression of the disease. The risks were immense; the patient's underdeveloped body was ill-prepared for such a trauma. Yet, the alternative was a slow and agonizing decline. The surgical team was assembled, and the operating room prepared.

The patient was wheeled into surgery, their tiny form dwarfed by the machinery and personnel surrounding them. The anesthesiologist carefully administered the anesthetic, mindful of the delicate balance required to keep the infant stable. As the surgeon made the first incision, there was a palpable tension in the room, a collective breath held in anticipation.

The damaged section of the intestine was identified and removed. It was a painstaking process, each movement precise and deliberate. The necrotic tissue was excised, and the remaining healthy bowel meticulously reconnected. Throughout the procedure, we monitored the patient's vital signs, adjusting fluids and medications to support the infant's tenuous hold on life.

Post-operatively, the patient was returned to the NICU, their condition critical but stable. The next 48 hours were crucial. We watched for signs of recovery, hoping for a reduction in abdominal distention and an improvement in blood gases. The patient remained on broad-spectrum antibiotics, and parenteral nutrition continued to provide the necessary sustenance.

Gradually, there were signs of improvement. The patient's abdomen softened, and the discoloration faded. Blood tests showed a decrease in inflammatory markers, and the metabolic acidosis began to resolve. Each small victory was a testament to the patient's tenacity and the skill of the medical team.

However, the road to recovery was fraught with challenges. The patient developed complications—a common occurrence in such fragile individuals. Infections, fluid imbalances, and feeding difficulties required constant vigilance and intervention. We adjusted treatments, administered additional medications, and provided meticulous care to address each new issue as it arose.

As days turned into weeks, the patient's condition stabilized. The feeding tube was gradually reintroduced, starting with minimal enteral nutrition to test the gut's functionality. Slowly, the patient began to tolerate small amounts of milk, a positive sign that the intestines were healing. The parenteral nutrition was tapered as enteral feeds increased, a delicate balance maintained to ensure the patient received adequate nutrition without overwhelming the recovering bowel.

Despite the progress, the patient remained vulnerable. Each day brought new challenges, and we remained vigilant, ever watchful for signs of relapse. The scars of NEC were both physical and metaphorical, a reminder of the precarious nature of life in the NICU. The patient's journey was a testament to the fortitude of the human spirit, a fragile yet unyielding force that defied the odds.

As the weeks turned into months, the patient's condition continued to improve. The transition from the NICU to the pediatric ward marked a significant milestone, a step towards a future that had once seemed uncertain. The patient's growth and development were closely monitored, ensuring that any lingering effects of NEC were promptly addressed.

Eventually, the day came when the patient was discharged from the hospital. It was a moment of profound relief and quiet triumph. The journey had been long and arduous, marked by moments of despair and glimmers of hope. The patient's survival was a testament to the collective efforts of the medical team and the indefatigable spirit of the tiny infant who had fought against all odds.

Reflecting on the experience, I was reminded of the delicate balance we strive to maintain in medicine. The patient's journey through NEC underscored the fragility of life and the resilience inherent in even the smallest and most vulnerable among us. It was a story of perseverance, of the indomitable will to survive, and of the unwavering dedication of those entrusted with the care of the most fragile lives.

In the end, the patient's recovery was not just a medical achievement but a profound affirmation of the human capacity to endure and overcome. It was a reminder that in the face of adversity, there is always hope, and that even in the darkest of times, the light of determination can guide us through.

As a doctor, I am often faced with the fragility of life and the limits of our abilities. But the story of the patient with Necrotizing Enterocolitis stands as a testament to the power of perseverance and the extraordinary resilience of the human spirit. It is a story that will stay with me always, a reminder of why we do what we do, and the profound impact we can have on the lives of those we are privileged to care for.

Chapter 13
KAT6A SYNDROME

AS A PEDIATRICIAN, I often encountered various medical conditions, but something about the patient's case was both unique and challenging. The patient, a small child of five, had been referred to me after a series of developmental concerns raised by their primary care physician. Upon entering the examination room, I was greeted by the anxious eyes of the patient's parents, who held their child close, seeking answers to the myriad questions that had plagued them for months.

The initial assessment was comprehensive. The patient exhibited notable delays in speech and motor skills, and there were distinct facial features that hinted at a genetic anomaly. The child's eyes, wide and expressive, seemed to communicate a world of thoughts trapped within a body that struggled to express them. The fingers were slender, and the overall build was slight. There was a certain fragility to the patient that was immediately apparent.

I began with a thorough review of the patient's medical history. The parents described a difficult infancy, marked by feeding problems and frequent hospital visits for unexplained fevers and infections. Growth had been slow, and milestones were consistently delayed. Despite these challenges, there was an undeniable spark in the patient's eyes, a silent determination that shone through even the toughest days.

After the physical examination and detailed history, I suspected a genetic disorder. The specific constellation of symptoms and physical features led me to consider KAT6A Syndrome, a rare and often underdiagnosed condition. To confirm this, I recommended a comprehensive genetic testing panel. The waiting period for the results was excruciating for the family, but it was necessary to obtain a definitive diagnosis.

Three weeks later, the results confirmed my suspicions: the patient had KAT6A Syndrome. This rare genetic disorder, caused by mutations in the KAT6A gene, explained the developmental delays, distinctive facial features, and other health issues. I sat with the family to explain the diagnosis, detailing the genetic underpinnings of the condition and what it meant for their child's future. I emphasized that while the syndrome presented significant challenges, there were steps we could take to manage the symptoms and improve the patient's quality of life.

The treatment plan was multi-faceted. It required a team approach, involving speech therapy, occupational therapy, physical therapy, and specialized educational interventions. I referred the patient to a speech therapist to address the communication difficulties. The therapist would work on enhancing verbal skills and, where necessary, introduce alternative communication methods, such as sign language or picture exchange systems.

Occupational therapy was crucial for improving fine motor skills and helping the patient achieve greater independence in daily activities. The occupational therapist would focus on activities that could enhance hand-eye coordination, dexterity, and self-care skills. Physical therapy was also essential to strengthen the patient's muscles, improve balance, and address any gait abnormalities.

In addition to these therapies, regular follow-ups with a geneticist and neurologist were scheduled to monitor the patient's progress and address any emerging issues. I also recommended consultations with a cardiologist and gastroenterologist, as KAT6A Syndrome could involve cardiac anomalies and gastrointestinal problems. The comprehensive care plan aimed to address the patient's medical, developmental, and educational needs holistically.

Over the next few months, the patient began to show signs of improvement. The speech therapist reported incremental progress in communication skills. The patient started using simple words and gestures more consistently, and there was a noticeable reduction in frustration during interactions. Occupational therapy sessions led to better fine motor control, and the patient could now handle small objects and perform basic self-care tasks with minimal assistance. Physical therapy also yielded positive results, with improved muscle tone and coordination.

Despite these advancements, the journey was far from easy. There were frequent setbacks, hospital visits for recurrent infections, and periods of stagnation in progress. The family remained deeply involved, attending every session and diligently practicing the exercises at home. Their unwavering dedication was inspiring and played a crucial role in the patient's development.

As months turned into years, the patient continued to make progress. By the age of seven, they were able to attend a specialized school that catered to children with developmental disabilities. The structured environment and tailored educational plans allowed the patient to thrive academically and socially. Teachers reported that the patient was eager to learn, showed curiosity, and had formed meaningful friendships with classmates.

However, the journey was not without its darker moments. The patient's health remained fragile, and there were several hospitalizations for pneumonia and other respiratory infections. Each episode was a stark reminder of the ongoing vulnerabilities and the need for vigilant medical care. The cardiologist monitored the patient closely for any signs of cardiac complications, but thankfully, none developed.

Around the age of ten, we faced a significant setback. The patient was diagnosed with epilepsy, a common comorbidity in individuals with KAT6A Syndrome. The seizures were initially mild but became more frequent and severe over time. Managing epilepsy required a delicate balance of medications and close monitoring to minimize side effects while controlling the seizures.

The introduction of antiepileptic drugs brought another layer of complexity to the treatment plan. The medications often caused drowsiness and affected the patient's cognitive function, impacting their ability to participate in therapy sessions and school activities. Adjusting the medication regimen was a continuous process, with the neurologist working tirelessly to find the optimal balance.

Despite these challenges, the patient's indomitable spirit shone through. They continued to engage in therapy, school, and social activities with an unyielding determination. By the age of twelve, the patient had achieved a level of independence that once seemed unattainable. They could communicate effectively using a combination of speech and gestures, perform most daily activities without assistance, and had a close-knit group of friends.

The family's support remained unwavering throughout this journey. Their home was a hub of love, encouragement, and tireless advocacy for the patient's needs. They navigated the complexities of the healthcare system with tenacity, ensuring that their child received the best possible care and opportunities for development.

As the patient approached adolescence, the focus of treatment shifted slightly. We continued to manage the epilepsy and monitor for any new health issues, but there was also a greater emphasis on preparing the patient for adulthood. This included life skills training, vocational education, and planning for future living arrangements. The goal was to equip the patient with the tools and support needed to lead a fulfilling and as independent a life as possible.

At sixteen, the patient faced another significant health challenge. They developed a severe respiratory infection that required prolonged hospitalization and intensive care. The infection exacerbated existing respiratory issues, and the patient's condition became critical. Despite the best efforts of the medical team, the patient's body struggled to fight the infection.

During this period, the family's presence was constant. They remained by the patient's side, providing comfort and reassurance. The medical team worked around the clock, employing every available treatment to stabilize the patient. It was a harrowing time, filled with uncertainty and fear.

Against all odds, the patient began to show signs of recovery. The infection gradually subsided, and the patient's condition stabilized. The road to recovery was long and arduous, but once again, the patient's remarkable fortitude came to the fore. Intensive rehabilitation followed, aimed at restoring the physical and functional abilities that had been compromised by the illness.

By the age of eighteen, the patient had made a remarkable recovery. They returned to their therapy and educational programs with renewed vigor. The experience had left its mark, but it also underscored the importance of resilience and the power of a supportive, loving family.

As the patient transitioned into adulthood, the focus of care continued to evolve. Vocational training programs helped the patient develop skills for future employment, and social services provided guidance on independent living arrangements. The patient's journey was a testament to the extraordinary impact of comprehensive, multidisciplinary care, and the unwavering support of family and community.

In reflecting on the patient's journey, I was struck by the remarkable progress made despite the significant challenges posed by KAT6A Syndrome. The initial diagnosis had been a turning point, setting in motion a comprehensive care plan that addressed the multifaceted needs of the patient. Each step of the journey was marked by incremental progress, setbacks, and a relentless pursuit of improvement.

The patient's story was a poignant reminder of the complexities and rewards of pediatric care. It underscored the importance of early diagnosis, personalized treatment plans, and the critical role of family and community support. While the journey was far from easy, it was filled with moments of triumph, growth, and a steadfast determination to overcome the odds.

In the end, the patient's story was one of hope and perseverance. It highlighted the incredible potential of individuals with KAT6A Syndrome to achieve meaningful progress and lead fulfilling lives. As a physician, it was an honor to be part of this journey, to witness the transformative power of comprehensive care, and to be reminded of the profound impact that a dedicated, multidisciplinary approach can have on the lives of patients and their families.

Chapter 14
IGA NEPHROPATHY

AS A NEPHROLOGIST, I was accustomed to dealing with complex and often disheartening cases. The patient, a middle-aged individual, had been referred to me due to persistent hematuria and proteinuria, symptoms that had raised red flags for their primary care physician.

The patient sat on the examination table, looking apprehensive yet hopeful. A detailed medical history was taken, revealing no significant past illnesses but a family history of hypertension and diabetes. The patient had noticed blood in their urine several times over the past few months, accompanied by occasional swelling in their legs and fatigue that was increasingly difficult to ignore.

After the initial assessment, I ordered a series of

tests, including blood work, urine analysis, and an ultrasound of the kidneys. The blood tests showed elevated creatinine and urea levels, indicating impaired kidney function. The urine analysis confirmed the presence of significant amounts of blood and protein. The ultrasound, however, did not reveal any structural abnormalities, making the diagnosis more challenging.

Given these findings, I decided that a kidney biopsy was necessary to pinpoint the exact cause of the patient's symptoms. The biopsy was performed under local anesthesia, and small samples of kidney tissue were extracted and sent to the pathology lab for analysis. A few days later, the results came back, confirming my suspicion: the patient had IgA Nephropathy.

IgA Nephropathy, also known as Berger's disease, is a condition where the antibody immunoglobulin A (IgA) builds up in the kidneys, leading to inflammation and damage. It is an autoimmune disorder with no known cure, and its progression can be unpredictable. Some patients manage well with minimal intervention, while others may progress to end-stage renal disease requiring dialysis or a kidney transplant.

The patient was informed of the diagnosis, and I began outlining the treatment plan. The primary goal was to slow the progression of the disease and manage the symptoms. We started with lifestyle modifications, advising the patient to reduce salt intake, follow a kidney-friendly diet, and maintain a healthy blood pressure. Antihypertensive medications, specifically angiotensin-converting enzyme (ACE) inhibitors, were prescribed to help control blood pressure and reduce proteinuria.

Regular follow-ups were scheduled to monitor the patient's condition closely. Initially, the patient responded well to the treatment. Blood pressure levels were maintained within the target range, and there was a slight reduction in proteinuria. The patient adhered to the dietary recommendations and reported feeling better overall. However, as months passed, the patient's kidney function continued to decline, albeit at a slower pace than before.

To manage the progressive nature of IgA Nephropathy, we introduced corticosteroids to the treatment regimen. Corticosteroids can suppress the immune system, reducing the inflammation caused by the IgA deposits. The patient was informed about the potential side effects, including weight gain, increased blood sugar levels, and a higher risk of infections. Despite these risks, the patient agreed to proceed, hopeful that this would help preserve kidney function.

The addition of corticosteroids initially showed promising results. The patient's proteinuria decreased significantly, and their kidney function stabilized. However, the side effects soon became apparent. The patient gained weight rapidly and experienced bouts of hyperglycemia, which required careful monitoring and adjustment of medications. Infections became more frequent, leading to hospitalizations for respiratory and urinary tract infections.

Throughout this period, the patient's spirits remained remarkably high. They continued to work, albeit on a reduced schedule, and engaged in various hobbies that brought them joy. Their family was supportive, attending appointments and ensuring the patient adhered to the treatment plan. It was evident that the patient had a robust support system, which played a crucial role in their ability to cope with the disease.

Despite our best efforts, the patient's kidney function began to decline more rapidly after two years. The creatinine and urea levels rose steadily, and the patient started experiencing symptoms of uremia, including nausea, fatigue, and a metallic taste in the mouth. The decision was made to prepare for renal replacement therapy. Given the patient's relatively young age and otherwise good health, a kidney transplant was considered the best option.

The patient was placed on the transplant waiting

list, and in the meantime, we initiated hemodialysis. The transition to dialysis was challenging. The patient struggled with the dietary restrictions and the time commitment required for thrice-weekly sessions. There were complications, including issues with the vascular access and episodes of hypotension during dialysis. Each setback was met with a mixture of frustration and determination.

After nearly a year on dialysis, the patient received a call that a suitable donor kidney was available. The transplant surgery was scheduled promptly, and the procedure went smoothly. The patient was monitored closely post-operatively for signs of rejection and infection. Immunosuppressive medications were started to prevent rejection of the new kidney.

The post-transplant period was marked by a roller-coaster of emotions and challenges. The patient's body initially accepted the new kidney well, and kidney function improved dramatically. However, the immunosuppressive therapy led to several complications, including opportunistic infections and metabolic imbalances. The patient developed diabetes as a side effect of the medications, requiring insulin therapy.

Despite these complications, the patient continued to persevere. Regular follow-ups with the transplant team and meticulous adherence to the medication regimen were essential in managing the new challenges. Over time, the frequency of infections decreased, and the patient's overall health began to stabilize. The new kidney functioned well, with creatinine levels returning to near-normal ranges.

The patient's life slowly began to regain a semblance of normalcy. They returned to work full-time, resumed their hobbies, and even took up new interests. The journey had been arduous, but the patient's determination and the support of their family had seen them through the darkest times. The experience had changed them, instilling a deeper appreciation for life and the small moments of joy it offered.

Years passed, and the patient continued to do well. Regular check-ups confirmed that the transplanted kidney was functioning optimally. The diabetes, while a challenge, was managed effectively with insulin and lifestyle modifications. The specter of IgA Nephropathy still lingered, as the disease could potentially recur in the transplanted kidney, but for now, the patient was enjoying a life free from the debilitating symptoms that once plagued them.

Reflecting on the patient's journey, I was reminded of the unpredictable nature of medicine. IgA Nephropathy is a disease that tests both the patient and the physician. It demands resilience, adaptability, and a strong support system. The patient's story was a testament to the advances in medical science and the indomitable spirit of those who face chronic illness with courage.

In the end, the patient's journey was one of triumph over adversity. While the road had been long and fraught with challenges, they emerged stronger and more appreciative of the life they fought so hard to preserve. Their story serves as an inspiration, a reminder that even in the face of a chronic and potentially devastating illness, there is hope and the possibility of a brighter future.

Chapter 15
GALACTOSEMIA

AS A PEDIATRICIAN with over twenty years of experience, I had seen a wide array of cases, but none left an imprint on my memory as deeply as the case of the infant with Galactosemia. This metabolic disorder was rare, and the intricacies involved in diagnosing and managing it made this particular case both challenging and poignant.

The patient came to us in the first few days of life, a period often marked by the sheer joy of new beginnings. However, for this family, those early days were fraught with concern. The infant, a seemingly healthy newborn at birth, began exhibiting alarming symptoms. Jaundice, poor feeding, vomiting, lethargy—these signs pointed to a deeper issue beyond the common ailments of newborns.

When the patient was brought into my clinic, my initial examination was guided by the urgency in the parents' eyes. Their baby was not thriving, and the typical causes like infections or birth complications had been ruled out. The infant's liver was enlarged, and there was noticeable weight loss, which compounded my concerns.

To pinpoint the cause, I ordered a series of blood tests. Among these was the galactosemia test, often included in newborn screening panels. Galactosemia, though rare, was a crucial condition to rule out because of its severe implications if left untreated. The test results came back confirming my suspicions: the patient had classic Galactosemia, a genetic disorder where the body is unable to process galactose properly due to a deficiency in the enzyme galactose-1-phosphate uridylyltransferase (GALT).

The confirmation of Galactosemia set into motion a series of immediate actions. The most critical was the immediate cessation of all milk products, including breast milk and formula that contained galactose. The patient was switched to a soy-based formula, which was free of galactose. This dietary intervention was the cornerstone of managing Galactosemia, as any galactose intake could lead to a toxic build-up in the body, causing severe complications like liver damage, intellectual disability, and even death.

As we transitioned the patient to the new formula, the symptoms gradually began to stabilize. The jaundice started to resolve, the vomiting ceased, and there was a noticeable improvement in energy levels and feeding patterns. However, the road ahead was still fraught with challenges. Galactosemia is not a condition that one simply grows out of; it requires lifelong dietary management and regular monitoring.

In the weeks that followed, I closely monitored the patient's progress. Regular blood tests were conducted to measure levels of galactose-1-phosphate, ensuring that the dietary restrictions were effective. The parents were educated extensively on the importance of adhering to the dietary guidelines and were provided with resources to manage this new aspect of their lives.

Despite the strict diet, there were still risks of long-term complications. We remained vigilant for signs of speech delays, learning difficulties, and issues with motor coordination. Early intervention programs and regular assessments by specialists were essential components of the patient's care plan.

As the patient grew, the diet remained strictly galactose-free. This meant that the family had to meticulously read food labels, avoid certain foods, and remain constantly vigilant. The burden on the parents was immense, but their dedication was unwavering. They attended every follow-up appointment, adhered to dietary guidelines, and engaged in support groups for families dealing with metabolic disorders.

By the time the patient reached preschool age, we noted some developmental delays, particularly in speech and fine motor skills. These were addressed with speech therapy and occupational therapy, which the patient responded to positively. Despite the challenges, there was a remarkable improvement in the patient's overall development and quality of life.

However, the specter of potential complications always loomed. As the patient entered school age, routine check-ups included assessments by neuropsychologists to monitor cognitive development. The risk of learning disabilities was high, but with early and ongoing interventions, we aimed to mitigate these impacts as much as possible.

During one particularly memorable follow-up visit, I noted how the patient, now a curious and spirited child, interacted with the world with a sense of determination that was both inspiring and heart-wrenching. The parents' unwavering commitment and the patient's intrinsic will to thrive were evident in every milestone achieved, no matter how small.

Over the years, the management of the patient's condition became more refined. Advances in medical research provided new insights into Galactosemia, and the patient benefited from the latest nutritional guidelines and therapeutic interventions. Genetic counseling was also a critical component of the patient's care, offering the family insights into the hereditary nature of the disorder and informing their decisions about future children.

Despite the meticulous care, adolescence brought a new set of challenges. The patient faced social and psychological hurdles, grappling with the restrictions imposed by their diet and the awareness of being different from peers. This period required not just medical oversight but also psychological support to help navigate the emotional landscape of growing up with a chronic condition.

At every stage, the patient's resilience in the face of adversity was striking. The family's unwavering support and the patient's adaptive spirit played a crucial role in managing the condition's impact. Regular check-ups continued to monitor liver function, cognitive development, and overall health. Each visit was a testament to the delicate balance maintained between medical intervention and the patient's determination.

As the patient transitioned into adulthood, the challenges evolved but the core approach remained the same: strict adherence to a galactose-free diet and regular medical monitoring. The focus shifted towards independence and self-management of the condition. The patient was educated on reading food labels, understanding nutritional information, and recognizing the signs of potential complications.

By this time, the patient had developed a deep understanding of their condition. They engaged actively in their healthcare, participated in discussions about their treatment plans, and even attended conferences on metabolic disorders. This proactive approach not only empowered the patient but also provided them with a sense of control over their life.

The transition to adulthood also brought considerations for long-term health and family planning. Genetic counseling sessions were revisited to discuss the implications of Galactosemia for future offspring. The patient's journey, from a fragile newborn to a self-assured adult, was marked by a series of adaptations, each requiring a nuanced approach to care and support.

Reflecting on the patient's journey, I realized that managing Galactosemia extended beyond medical intervention. It encompassed education, emotional support, and an unwavering commitment from both the healthcare team and the family. Each phase of the patient's life brought new challenges, but also new triumphs, each small victory a testament to the indomitable human spirit.

In the end, the patient's story was one of survival, adaptation, and continuous learning. It highlighted the importance of early diagnosis, rigorous treatment, and the critical role of a supportive environment. Through the combined efforts of medical science, family dedication, and the patient's own determination, the battle against Galactosemia was met with remarkable fortitude.

This case reminded me of the profound impact of holistic care, where treating the condition also meant supporting the individual and their family. It underscored the importance of staying updated with medical advances, providing compassionate care, and recognizing the strength within each patient to overcome the challenges posed by their condition.

As I continued my practice, the lessons from this case stayed with me, guiding my approach to each new patient. It reinforced my belief in the power of early intervention, comprehensive care, and the extraordinary capacity of patients and their families to navigate the complexities of life with chronic conditions. The patient's journey was not just a medical case but a story of enduring spirit and unwavering support, a story that would continue to inspire and inform my work for years to come.

Chapter 16
ELLIS-VAN CREVELD SYNDROME

THE FIRST TIME I saw the patient was during my residency in pediatric medicine. The patient, a newborn, was brought to our clinic by anxious parents who had already sensed something was not quite right. As the on-call pediatrician, I conducted the initial examination, unaware that this encounter would leave an indelible mark on my medical career.

The patient's physical features immediately drew my attention. The short limbs, extra fingers, and a slightly sunken chest were indicative of a genetic disorder. As I examined the patient, I noticed a heart murmur, which further raised my suspicions. I knew then that we were dealing with something beyond the typical congenital abnormalities. The patient's breathing was shallow, and there were slight cyanotic tinges around the lips, indicating potential cardiovascular complications.

Ellis-Van Creveld syndrome (EVC) was my initial suspicion, given the patient's phenotypic presentation. EVC is a rare genetic disorder characterized by skeletal dysplasia, heart defects, and, often, dental anomalies. It is also known for causing a form of dwarfism, with affected individuals having shorter limbs compared to their torso.

To confirm my suspicion, I ordered a series of diagnostic tests. Radiographs were taken to examine the skeletal structure, and an echocardiogram was performed to assess the extent of any cardiac anomalies. Additionally, genetic testing was essential to confirm the diagnosis definitively.

The radiographs revealed the classic features of Ellis-Van Creveld syndrome: short ribs, postaxial polydactyly (extra fingers), and shortened long bones. The echocardiogram showed a common atrium, a significant congenital heart defect associated with EVC, where the atria of the heart are not properly separated. This explained the heart murmur and cyanosis I had observed earlier. Genetic testing confirmed the presence of mutations in the EVC1 and EVC2 genes, validating my clinical diagnosis.

With the diagnosis confirmed, the challenge was now to manage and treat the patient's condition effectively. Ellis-Van Creveld syndrome is a lifelong condition with no cure, and treatment is primarily focused on managing symptoms and improving quality of life. The patient required a multidisciplinary approach involving cardiologists, orthopedic surgeons, and dental specialists.

The most urgent concern was the cardiac defect. The common atrium could lead to severe complications if not addressed promptly. The patient was referred to a pediatric cardiologist who recommended surgical correction. The procedure was high-risk due to the patient's small size and fragile state, but it was necessary to improve the patient's chances of survival.

The surgery was scheduled, and in the interim, we focused on managing the patient's respiratory issues. Frequent monitoring and oxygen supplementation were necessary to ensure that the patient's oxygen levels remained stable. Nutritional support was also critical, as infants with EVC often have difficulty feeding due to their dental anomalies and oral structure.

On the day of the surgery, there was a palpable tension in the air. The operating room team was prepared for the complexities that lay ahead. I watched as the anesthesiologist carefully administered the anesthesia, mindful of the patient's delicate condition. The cardiac surgeon began the intricate procedure to correct the heart defect.

The hours passed slowly, each one laden with the weight of uncertainty. Finally, the surgeon emerged, his expression a mixture of exhaustion and cautious optimism. The surgery had been successful, but the patient was not out of the woods yet. The next 48 hours would be critical as we monitored for any signs of complications.

Post-surgery, the patient was transferred to the neonatal intensive care unit (NICU). The patient's recovery was closely monitored by a team of dedicated nurses and doctors. The patient remained intubated for several days, gradually showing signs of improvement. The cyanosis began to diminish, and the patient's breathing became more stable.

As the days turned into weeks, the patient continued to make slow but steady progress. The intubation was eventually removed, and the patient was able to breathe independently, a significant milestone in the recovery process. The patient's parents were visibly relieved, though the road ahead remained long and uncertain.

Orthopedic interventions were the next focus. The

patient's short limbs and polydactyly required surgical correction to improve functionality. The orthopedic surgeon outlined a series of procedures that would be performed over the next few years to address these issues. The first surgery was to remove the extra fingers, which would help the patient develop better hand function.

The recovery from the orthopedic surgery was less fraught with complications than the cardiac surgery, though it was not without its challenges. The patient was fitted with tiny casts, and physical therapy was initiated to ensure proper healing and development of motor skills. Regular follow-ups with the orthopedic team became a part of the patient's routine.

Dental issues were also a significant concern. EVC often results in abnormal tooth development, and the patient was no exception. Early intervention by a pediatric dentist was crucial to manage these issues. The patient was fitted with special dental appliances to aid in feeding and later in speech development. These appliances needed to be regularly adjusted as the patient grew.

Over the next few years, the patient's medical journey was marked by frequent hospital visits, surgeries, and therapies. Despite these challenges, the patient demonstrated an extraordinary capacity to endure and adapt. The parents were unwavering in their support, navigating the complexities of the medical system with determination.

At the age of five, the patient underwent a comprehensive evaluation to assess overall development. The orthopedic surgeries had significantly improved limb functionality, and the cardiac surgery had corrected the major heart defect. However, the patient still faced several ongoing challenges, including dental issues and the need for additional orthopedic interventions.

Regular physical therapy sessions had helped the patient develop gross motor skills, though fine motor skills remained a work in progress. The patient's cognitive development was within normal limits, a positive sign given the initial concerns about potential neurological involvement.

As the patient entered school, the social implications of EVC became more apparent. The patient's short stature and physical differences were noticeable, and the family worked closely with educators to ensure an inclusive and supportive environment. The patient's peers, curious but accepting, gradually became accustomed to these differences.

The patient's medical team continued to monitor for any new complications. Regular cardiac evaluations were essential to ensure that the heart remained stable. The orthopedic team planned additional surgeries to address growth-related issues, and the dental team continued to manage the patient's oral health.

By the age of ten, the patient had undergone multiple surgeries and interventions. Each procedure brought new challenges, but also new milestones. The patient's ability to walk and perform daily activities improved significantly. Dental appliances had been replaced by more permanent solutions, allowing for better nutrition and oral health.

The patient's adolescence brought its own set of challenges. The typical growth spurts and hormonal changes were complicated by the underlying condition. The patient faced social and emotional hurdles, grappling with self-esteem and body image issues. Psychological support became an integral part of the care plan, helping the patient navigate these turbulent years.

Despite these challenges, the patient showed remarkable strength. Academic achievements were a source of pride, and the patient pursued interests and hobbies with enthusiasm. The medical team continued to provide comprehensive care, addressing each new issue with the same dedication and expertise as before.

As the patient reached adulthood, the focus shifted to long-term management and independence. The patient had developed a thorough understanding of their condition and actively participated in medical decisions. Regular check-ups, physical therapy, and dental care remained essential components of the care plan.

The patient's transition to adult care was carefully managed to ensure continuity. Specialists in adult congenital heart disease, orthopedics, and dentistry took over the patient's care. The patient adapted well to this transition, demonstrating the resilience and determination that had defined their journey from the beginning.

The patient's life was marked by a series of triumphs and setbacks, each contributing to a story of remarkable fortitude. The congenital heart defect had been successfully managed, though regular monitoring was still necessary. The orthopedic interventions had significantly improved mobility, though the patient continued to require occasional surgeries to address growth-related issues.

The patient's dental health had been a constant challenge, but with ongoing care, the issues were manageable. Psychological support remained a vital aspect of the patient's care, helping navigate the complexities of living with a chronic condition.

Looking back on the patient's journey, I was struck

by the sheer determination that defined each step. The patient's ability to endure and adapt to the challenges posed by Ellis-Van Creveld syndrome was nothing short of extraordinary. The medical team's collaborative efforts had significantly improved the patient's quality of life, but it was the patient's own strength and tenacity that truly made the difference.

The patient's story is a testament to the advances in medical science and the importance of a comprehensive, multidisciplinary approach to care. It also underscores the vital role of support systems, both familial and medical, in managing chronic conditions. Each member of the patient's care team contributed to a tapestry of care that supported and nurtured the patient through the years.

In my career as a pediatrician, the patient's case remains one of the most profound examples of the impact of dedicated, compassionate care. It taught me the importance of looking beyond the medical charts and understanding the human experience of those we treat. The patient's journey with Ellis-Van Creveld syndrome is a story of courage, endurance, and an unwavering will to thrive despite the odds.

In conclusion, the patient's life, though fraught with medical challenges, was also filled with moments of joy, achievement, and hope. The patient did not merely survive but lived, carving out a path that defied the limitations imposed by a rare genetic disorder. The journey was long and often arduous, but it was also a testament to the resilience of the human spirit and the profound impact of compassionate, comprehensive medical care.

Chapter 17
CAMURATI-ENGELMANN DISEASE

THE PATIENT first came to my attention on a dreary Monday morning, as I shuffled through a stack of medical charts and X-rays in the dimly lit office of the hospital. Their case file was unremarkable at first glance, buried beneath the routine ailments and familiar maladies that comprised my daily workload. Yet, as I flipped through the initial pages, a peculiar pattern in the symptoms caught my eye. The patient, a young adult, had been suffering from an inexplicable and progressive pain in their limbs, coupled with a noticeable thickening of the bones.

My curiosity piqued, I decided to delve deeper into the patient's history. Over the next few days, I pored over their medical records, noting the frequent visits to various clinics and hospitals, the endless rounds of inconclusive tests, and the growing frustration etched in the notes of previous physicians. The symptoms had first appeared in late adolescence, insidious and subtle, manifesting as intermittent discomfort and fatigue. Over the years, the pain had escalated, becoming a constant, debilitating presence that resisted all conventional treatments.

A thorough examination was imperative. When the patient arrived for their appointment, I could see the weariness in their eyes, a reflection of the relentless ordeal they had endured. Their gait was unsteady, each step a visible effort, and they carried the weight of chronic pain with a stoic determination. As I conducted a physical examination, I observed the characteristic signs: the pronounced thickening of the long bones in the arms and legs, the abnormal gait, and the tenderness in the affected areas. These were hallmarks of a rare and enigmatic condition—Camurati-Engelmann Disease.

Camurati-Engelmann Disease, or progressive diaphyseal dysplasia, is a genetic disorder characterized by abnormal bone formation and remodeling. It primarily affects the long bones, leading to their thickening and causing severe pain and weakness. The disease is hereditary, linked to mutations in the TGFB1 gene, which plays a crucial role in bone development and maintenance. Despite its genetic origins, the disease's progression and severity can vary widely among individuals, presenting a formidable challenge for diagnosis and treatment.

The diagnosis, while offering a semblance of clarity, also brought with it a profound sense of trepidation. There was no cure for Camurati-Engelmann Disease, and the management of its symptoms required a nuanced and multidisciplinary approach. My first step was to assemble a team of specialists, including geneticists, orthopedists, and pain management experts, to develop a comprehensive treatment plan tailored to the patient's needs.

Genetic testing confirmed the presence of the TGFB1 mutation, providing a definitive diagnosis. The patient's genetic counselor explained the hereditary nature of the disease, offering insights into its transmission and potential implications for future generations. This revelation added an emotional dimension to the patient's struggle, intertwining their physical pain with concerns about their family and descendants.

Pain management became our immediate priority. The patient had already tried a myriad of analgesics and anti-inflammatory medications, with limited success. We explored alternative therapies, including nerve blocks and physical therapy, to alleviate the chronic discomfort. A regimen of corticosteroids was introduced to reduce inflammation and slow the progression of bone thickening. However, the side effects of long-term steroid use posed additional risks, necessitating careful monitoring and dosage adjustments.

Orthopedic intervention was another critical aspect of the treatment plan. The excessive bone growth in the patient's limbs had begun to compromise their mobility and quality of life. Surgical options, such as decompression and resection of the thickened bone, were considered to relieve pressure on the surrounding tissues and nerves. These procedures, while offering potential relief, carried significant risks and required meticulous planning and execution.

Throughout this journey, the patient's perseverance was remarkable. They adhered to the treatment regimen with unwavering dedication, attending regular physical therapy sessions and diligently following medical advice. The physical therapist worked to strengthen the muscles around the affected bones, enhancing stability and reducing the strain on the skeletal system. These sessions, though arduous, provided incremental improvements, offering a glimmer of hope in an otherwise bleak landscape.

The patient's emotional well-being was another

crucial consideration. The chronic pain and physical limitations imposed by Camurati-Engelmann Disease had taken a toll on their mental health. A psychologist was brought in to provide counseling and support, helping the patient navigate the emotional challenges of living with a chronic, incurable condition. This holistic approach aimed to address not only the physical symptoms but also the psychological impact of the disease.

Over the following months, the patient's condition fluctuated. There were periods of relative stability, where the pain was manageable, and mobility was slightly improved. These brief respites were often followed by exacerbations, episodes of intense pain and increased bone thickening that undermined the progress we had made. Each setback was a stark reminder of the relentless nature of the disease, yet the patient faced these challenges with a quiet fortitude, a testament to their enduring spirit.

Despite our best efforts, the disease continued its inexorable march. The patient's mobility became increasingly impaired, and the pain more pervasive. We explored experimental treatments, including bisphosphonates and monoclonal antibodies, which showed promise in early-stage trials. These therapies aimed to regulate bone metabolism and inhibit abnormal bone growth, offering a potential breakthrough in managing the disease. However, their efficacy remained uncertain, and the long-term effects were unknown.

As the years passed, the patient's condition reached a critical juncture. The thickening of the bones had progressed to the point where surgical intervention was no longer viable. The pain, once a background hum, had become a constant, unrelenting companion. The patient was confined to a wheelchair, their body a prisoner of the disease that had ravaged their bones and sapped their strength.

Palliative care became our focus, shifting from curative attempts to improving the patient's quality of life in their remaining days. Pain management was intensified, employing a combination of opioids and adjuvant therapies to provide relief. The patient's psychological support network was fortified, ensuring they had access to counseling and emotional support.

The patient's family, who had been a steadfast source of support throughout the ordeal, rallied around them. Their home was adapted to accommodate the patient's needs, with modifications to enhance accessibility and comfort. Hospice care was arranged, providing specialized medical and emotional support as the patient's condition deteriorated.

In the final months, the patient's decline was rapid.

The pain, despite our best efforts, became unmanageable, and their physical condition deteriorated. The disease had taken its toll, eroding their body and spirit. Yet, even in these darkest moments, there was a palpable sense of acceptance, a quiet acknowledgment of the inevitable.

The patient passed away peacefully in their sleep, surrounded by family and enveloped in love. Their journey had been one of immense struggle and profound courage, a testament to the human spirit's capacity to endure in the face of insurmountable odds. Their death, while a poignant loss, brought an end to the suffering that had defined their final years.

In the aftermath, I reflected on the journey we had shared. The patient's battle with Camurati-Engelmann Disease had been a harsh reminder of the limitations of modern medicine and the unpredictable nature of genetic disorders. It underscored the importance of a holistic approach to treatment, one that addresses not only the physical symptoms but also the emotional and psychological impacts of chronic illness.

The case also highlighted the need for continued research and innovation in the field of genetic diseases. Camurati-Engelmann Disease, like many rare disorders, remained a challenging frontier, requiring a deeper understanding of its pathophysiology and the development of targeted therapies. The patient's journey served as a catalyst for further investigation, inspiring a renewed commitment to unraveling the mysteries of this enigmatic disease.

In the end, the patient's legacy was one of courage and determination. Their story, marked by relentless pain and unyielding fortitude, left an indelible mark on all who had the privilege of caring for them. It was a reminder of the profound impact that a single life can have, even in the face of overwhelming adversity. The patient's journey, though fraught with suffering, was a testament to the enduring power of the human spirit, a beacon of hope for all who continue to fight against the odds.

As a physician, I was profoundly changed by this experience. It reinforced my commitment to compassionate care and the importance of supporting patients not only as medical cases but as individuals with unique stories and struggles. The patient's journey with Camurati-Engelmann Disease was a poignant reminder of the fragility of life and the enduring strength of the human spirit, a lesson that would stay with me for the rest of my career.

Chapter 18
ABETALIPOPROTEINEMIA

I FIRST MET the patient during a routine checkup at the clinic. They were a young individual, barely out of their teenage years, with an air of fatigue that seemed disproportionate to their age. They complained of chronic fatigue, difficulty in seeing at night, and frequent episodes of diarrhea. Their skin had a peculiar paleness, and their gait was slightly unsteady, suggestive of a deeper underlying issue.

As a physician, I had encountered various rare diseases over my career, but nothing quite prepared me for what lay ahead with this patient. The initial blood tests were perplexing. The patient's cholesterol levels were abnormally low, something quite unusual for someone their age and general health status. Additionally, there was a significant deficiency in fat-soluble vitamins, particularly vitamins A, D, E, and K. These initial findings prompted me to delve deeper.

I recommended a series of more specialized tests, including a lipid profile and genetic testing. While waiting for the results, I started the patient on a regimen of vitamin supplements, particularly focusing on the fat-soluble vitamins they were deficient in. The goal was to mitigate some of their symptoms and stabilize their condition while we investigated further.

The results, when they arrived, were both illuminating and daunting. The genetic tests confirmed my growing suspicion: the patient had Abetalipoproteinemia, a rare genetic disorder that impairs the body's ability to absorb dietary fats, cholesterol, and certain vitamins. This disorder is caused by mutations in the MTTP gene, which is responsible for producing a protein essential for the proper assembly and secretion of lipoproteins containing apolipoprotein B.

Abetalipoproteinemia is an autosomal recessive disorder, meaning both copies of the gene in each cell have mutations. This explained the patient's symptoms: the chronic fatigue, the night blindness, the neurological symptoms, and the gastrointestinal issues. Their body simply couldn't process fats and fat-soluble vitamins properly, leading to a cascade of health problems.

Understanding the gravity of the situation, I called

the patient's family to explain the diagnosis. It was a difficult conversation, laden with medical jargon that needed careful translation into comprehensible terms. The patient's condition was life-altering and would require a multifaceted treatment approach. There was no cure, only management of symptoms and prevention of complications.

The cornerstone of managing Abetalipoproteinemia is dietary modification. I referred the patient to a nutritionist who specialized in rare metabolic disorders. Together, we devised a diet plan that was extremely low in fat but rich in essential fatty acids from sources that the patient could tolerate. Medium-chain triglycerides (MCTs) were incorporated into their diet as these can be absorbed directly into the bloodstream, bypassing the normal fat absorption pathway which is defective in Abetalipoproteinemia.

In addition to the dietary changes, I prescribed high doses of fat-soluble vitamins A, D, E, and K. These vitamins are crucial for various bodily functions, and their deficiency was contributing significantly to the patient's symptoms. Vitamin A was particularly important for their vision problems, while vitamin E was essential for preventing neurological damage.

The patient's treatment regimen also included regular blood tests to monitor their vitamin levels and overall health. Given the nature of their disorder, they were prone to developing complications such as retinal degeneration, neuropathy, and muscle weakness. Regular monitoring was vital to catch any issues early and adjust their treatment as necessary.

As months turned into years, the patient became a frequent visitor to the clinic. Their progress was a testament to their remarkable fortitude. The dietary modifications and vitamin supplementation brought noticeable improvements. The night blindness reduced significantly, and their overall energy levels improved. They even reported fewer episodes of diarrhea and a better quality of life.

However, the journey was not without its challenges. The patient had to adhere strictly to their dietary restrictions, which was no small feat. Social gatherings and meals became a source of anxiety, as they constantly had to ensure their food was prepared in a way that met their dietary needs. The psychological burden of living with a chronic, rare disease was immense. They faced moments of frustration and isolation, but they persevered, driven by an unwavering determination to maintain their health.

Regular neurological assessments were an integral part of their follow-up. Abetalipoproteinemia can lead to progressive neurological deterioration, and I was keen to catch any signs of this early. The patient's reflexes and coordination were closely monitored, and while there were occasional setbacks, they showed an admirable ability to adapt and manage their symptoms.

One of the more concerning developments occurred a few years into their treatment. Despite the high doses of vitamin E, the patient began to exhibit signs of peripheral neuropathy. They experienced numbness and tingling in their extremities, and their gait became more unsteady. This was a stark reminder of the relentless nature of their condition and the limitations of current medical interventions.

To address this, I collaborated with a neurologist who had experience with neurodegenerative disorders. We adjusted the patient's vitamin E dosage and introduced physical therapy to help maintain their muscle strength and coordination. The physical therapy sessions became a crucial part of their routine, providing not only physical benefits but also a sense of agency over their condition.

As time passed, the patient's resilience was tested further. They developed scoliosis, a common complication in individuals with Abetalipoproteinemia due to muscle weakness. The curvature of their spine required orthopedic intervention, and they underwent a surgical procedure to correct it. The recovery was arduous, but the patient faced it with the same tenacity they had shown throughout their treatment.

In the years that followed, the patient's condition stabilized to a degree. Their adherence to the dietary regimen and vitamin supplementation paid off, and they managed to avoid many of the more severe complications associated with Abetalipoproteinemia. They found a balance that allowed them to lead a relatively normal life, albeit with constant vigilance.

Their journey was a profound reminder of the challenges faced by those with rare diseases. Every aspect of their life was influenced by their condition, from their diet to their social interactions to their long-term health. Yet, they navigated these challenges with an extraordinary spirit.

Ultimately, the patient's story did not culminate in a miraculous cure. Abetalipoproteinemia remains a lifelong condition without a definitive cure. However, through meticulous management and an indomitable spirit, the patient achieved a quality of life that many might have deemed impossible at the outset. They adapted, they endured, and they found ways to thrive despite the constant presence of their condition.

As a doctor, I was humbled by the experience. Treating someone with Abetalipoproteinemia required more than just medical knowledge; it demanded empathy, creativity, and a deep commitment to the patient's well-being. It reinforced the importance of a holistic approach to healthcare, one that considers not just the physical but also the emotional and psychological aspects of living with a chronic condition.

The patient's journey with Abetalipoproteinemia was one of constant adaptation and unwavering fortitude. Their story is a testament to the strength of the human spirit in the face of adversity and the potential of modern medicine to improve lives, even when a cure remains out of reach. Through meticulous management and relentless perseverance, the patient was able to carve out a life marked not by their disease, but by their courage and determination.

Chapter 19
TAKOTSUBO CARDIOMYOPATHY
(BROKEN HEART SYNDROME)

TAKOTSUBO CARDIOMYOPATHY, often referred to as "broken heart syndrome," is a condition that mimics a heart attack but is precipitated by extreme emotional or physical stress. I encountered a particularly memorable case of this condition during my tenure at the hospital. This is the story of one such patient.

The patient was admitted to the emergency room on a stormy evening, clutching their chest and gasping for breath. The signs were ominous: crushing chest pain, shortness of breath, and an overwhelming sense of dread. Initial examinations suggested a myocardial infarction, but something about the patient's demeanor and presentation suggested there might be more to the story.

Upon arrival, the patient was immediately taken for an electrocardiogram (ECG). The results showed significant ST-segment elevation, a hallmark of a heart attack. However, there were subtle differences in the ECG patterns that raised my suspicion. The absence of reciprocal changes and the presence of deep T-wave inversions in the anterior leads suggested a different pathology.

Further investigation was warranted, and we proceeded with a blood test to measure cardiac enzymes. Elevated troponin levels confirmed myocardial injury, yet the pattern did not fit neatly into the typical presentation of a coronary artery blockage. The patient's angiogram revealed clean coronary arteries, which was unexpected. This crucial finding pointed towards a diagnosis of Takotsubo Cardiomyopathy.

Takotsubo Cardiomyopathy, named for the Japanese octopus trap it resembles due to the ballooning of the left ventricle, is an unusual condition. It is typically triggered by severe emotional or physical stress, leading to a temporary weakening of the heart muscle. In this case, the patient had experienced a significant personal loss, which had likely precipitated the episode.

With the diagnosis confirmed, our focus shifted to

treatment. The primary goal was to stabilize the patient and support their heart function while it recovered. The initial approach involved administering medications to manage the symptoms and prevent complications. We started the patient on beta-blockers to reduce the heart's workload and improve its efficiency. Angiotensin-converting enzyme (ACE) inhibitors were also prescribed to help the heart muscle recover and prevent further damage.

The patient was closely monitored in the intensive care unit. Continuous ECG monitoring was essential to detect any arrhythmias, which are common in Takotsubo Cardiomyopathy. The patient was also given diuretics to manage fluid retention and ease the strain on the heart. Despite these measures, the patient's condition remained precarious during the first few days of hospitalization.

The patient's emotional state was a critical aspect of their recovery. Psychological support was just as important as medical intervention. A psychiatrist was consulted to provide counseling and help the patient navigate their grief. The connection between mind and body was evident in this case, and addressing the emotional turmoil was essential for holistic healing.

Gradually, the patient's condition began to improve.

The supportive care, both medical and psychological, started to show positive effects. The heart's function, assessed through echocardiograms, showed signs of recovery. The left ventricle, which had ballooned out during the acute phase, began to return to its normal shape and size.

Despite the progress, the patient faced several challenges. The path to recovery from Takotsubo Cardiomyopathy is not always straightforward. Episodes of heart failure, arrhythmias, and even thromboembolic events are possible complications. The patient experienced intermittent arrhythmias, which required careful management with antiarrhythmic drugs.

One evening, the patient experienced a sudden onset of ventricular tachycardia, a life-threatening arrhythmia. The rapid, erratic heartbeats caused a sharp drop in blood pressure, leading to syncope. Emergency measures were implemented swiftly. The patient was defibrillated to restore a normal heart rhythm and was immediately transferred back to the intensive care unit for closer monitoring. This incident underscored the fragile nature of their recovery.

In the ICU, the patient was placed on intravenous antiarrhythmics and continuous cardiac monitoring. The episode of ventricular tachycardia had been a stark reminder of the potential dangers associated with Takotsubo Cardiomyopathy. Despite the initial scare, the patient stabilized once again.

As the weeks passed, the patient's condition gradually improved. The frequency and severity of arrhythmias decreased, and the heart's function continued to normalize. Repeat echocardiograms showed significant improvement in the ejection fraction, indicating a recovering heart muscle. This progress allowed us to gradually wean the patient off some of the medications.

Throughout this period, the patient's psychological state remained a crucial aspect of care. Regular sessions with the psychiatrist helped the patient process their grief and develop coping mechanisms. The integration of psychological support into the treatment plan was a key factor in the patient's overall improvement.

By the third week of hospitalization, the patient was stable enough to be transferred to a regular ward. The transition from intensive care to a general medical ward marked a significant milestone in their recovery. The patient was no longer dependent on continuous cardiac monitoring, and the risk of acute complications had diminished.

In the general ward, the focus shifted towards rehabilitation and preparation for discharge. The patient participated in a cardiac rehabilitation program, which included supervised physical activity and education about heart health. This program was designed to gradually rebuild physical strength and stamina, as well as to provide the patient with the tools needed to manage their condition in the long term.

The patient's recovery journey was not just about physical healing but also about regaining confidence in their own body. The cardiac rehabilitation program played a vital role in this process. The patient began with light exercises, such as walking on a treadmill, under close supervision. Over time, the intensity of the exercises was gradually increased, helping to rebuild cardiovascular fitness.

Education was another important component of the rehabilitation program. The patient attended sessions that covered topics such as heart-healthy diet, stress management, and the importance of adherence to medications. These sessions were designed to empower the patient with knowledge and skills to prevent future cardiac events.

By the time the patient was ready for discharge, their heart function had significantly improved. Echocardiograms showed that the left ventricle had returned to its normal shape, and the ejection fraction was within the normal range. The patient's recovery from Takotsubo Cardiomyopathy was remarkable, but it was also a testament to the comprehensive care they had received.

Before discharge, the patient was provided with a detailed plan for follow-up care. This included regular visits to the cardiologist to monitor heart function, as well as ongoing psychological support. The patient was also advised to continue the cardiac rehabilitation program on an outpatient basis.

Leaving the hospital was both a moment of triumph and a new beginning for the patient. The journey of recovery from Takotsubo Cardiomyopathy is a long one, and it requires ongoing attention to both physical and emotional health. The patient was encouraged to remain vigilant about their heart health and to seek help promptly if they experienced any new symptoms.

In the months following discharge, the patient adhered to their follow-up care plan diligently. Regular visits to the cardiologist showed continued improvement in heart function, and there were no further episodes of arrhythmias. The patient also continued to engage in the cardiac rehabilitation program, which helped them maintain physical fitness and confidence in their recovery.

The patient's emotional well-being also improved significantly. The regular sessions with the psychiatrist helped them process their grief and develop healthy coping mechanisms. Over time, the emotional scars began to heal, and the patient found new ways to cope with stress.

Looking back on this case, it was a profound reminder of the intricate link between emotional and physical health. Takotsubo Cardiomyopathy, often precipitated by intense emotional stress, underscores the importance of a holistic approach to patient care. The patient's recovery was a testament to the effectiveness of combining medical treatment with psychological support.

This case also highlighted the need for awareness about Takotsubo Cardiomyopathy. While it is less common than traditional myocardial infarction, it is a significant condition that requires prompt diagnosis and appropriate management. The lessons learned from this case have influenced my approach to patient care, emphasizing the need to look beyond the physical symptoms and consider the emotional context as well.

In conclusion, the patient's journey through Takotsubo Cardiomyopathy was a challenging yet enlightening experience. It was a testament to the power of comprehensive care and the importance of addressing both physical and emotional health. The patient's eventual recovery, marked by the normalization of heart function and improved emotional well-being, was a triumph of medical science and compassionate care.

Chapter 20
LANDAU KLEFFNER SYNDROME

AS A NEUROLOGIST with decades of experience, I have encountered countless patients, each with their own unique story and challenges. However, there is one case that has left an indelible mark on my career and my life: the patient with Landau Kleffner Syndrome (LKS).

I first met the patient when they were just a young child, brought to my office by their parents who were desperate for answers. They described a once vibrant and talkative child who had gradually withdrawn into a world of silence, their language skills deteriorating rapidly. The parents spoke of the heartbreak they felt watching their child slip away, unable to communicate or connect with the world around them.

During the initial examination, I observed a child

who appeared alert and engaged, but struggled to express themselves. Their eyes darted around the room, searching for a way to convey their thoughts and feelings, but the words remained trapped inside their mind.

I suspected LKS, a rare neurological disorder that affects the brain's ability to process and understand language, often accompanied by epileptic seizures. To confirm my diagnosis, I ordered a series of tests, including an EEG and an MRI.

The results were conclusive, and I found myself faced with the daunting task of explaining the nature of LKS to the patient's family. I described how the disorder would impact their child's language development and the long road ahead filled with therapy, medication, and uncertainty.

The parents listened intently, their faces etched with a mixture of fear, confusion, and determination. They asked questions, seeking to understand every aspect of their child's condition and what they could do to help. I admired their strength and resilience in the face of such a devastating diagnosis.

We wasted no time in starting treatment, beginning with anti-epileptic medications to control the patient's seizures. The child responded positively at first, with a noticeable reduction in seizure frequency and severity.

However, the language deficits persisted, and progress was painstakingly slow.

In addition to medication, we implemented a multidisciplinary approach to therapy, involving speech and language pathologists, occupational therapists, and special education teachers. The goal was to help the patient regain their lost language skills and develop alternative methods of communication.

Months turned into years, and the patient's journey was marked by a series of highs and lows. There were moments of breakthrough, where a word or phrase would suddenly emerge from the silence, giving us all a glimmer of hope. But these moments were often fleeting, and the disorder's grip on the child's language abilities remained strong.

Throughout this time, I watched as the family's determination and love for their child never wavered. They celebrated every small victory, cherishing each hard-won word or gesture. They became fierce advocates for their child, tirelessly researching new treatments and therapies, and connecting with other families affected by LKS.

As the years passed, the patient's condition stabilized, but the language deficits remained significant. The seizures were mostly under control, but the damage to the language centers of the brain was extensive. The once bright-eyed child had grown into a teenager, navigating a world that often misunderstood and underestimated them.

Despite the challenges imposed by LKS, the patient found ways to express themselves and connect with others. They developed a unique sign language with their family, using gestures and facial expressions to convey their thoughts and emotions. They also learned to use assistive technology, such as communication boards and speech-generating devices, to communicate their needs and desires.

I continued to monitor the patient's progress, adjusting medications and therapy plans as needed. We explored new treatment options, including experimental drugs and surgical interventions, but none proved to be the miracle cure we hoped for.

As the patient entered adulthood, I reflected on the incredible journey we had taken together. LKS had taken so much from them, robbing them of the ability to communicate through spoken language. But it had also revealed an inner strength and determination that was truly awe-inspiring. The patient and their family had faced unimaginable challenges, but they had never given up hope.

In the end, the patient's story was not one of a miraculous recovery or a return to a life before LKS.

Instead, it was a testament to the power of the human spirit to adapt, persevere, and find joy in the face of adversity. The patient may not have regained their language skills, but they had found other ways to express themselves and connect with the world around them.

As a doctor, I had learned invaluable lessons from this patient and their family. They had taught me the true meaning of courage, love, and unwavering commitment. They had shown me that even in the darkest of times, there is always a reason to hope and to keep fighting.

Today, the patient continues to live with LKS, but they refuse to be defined by it. They have built a life filled with love, laughter, and purpose, surrounded by a family and community that supports and understands them. They have become an inspiration to others facing similar challenges, a shining example of what is possible when we refuse to give up.

As I look back on my career and the countless patients I have had the privilege to treat, this one stands out as a true embodiment of the indomitable human spirit. They may not have conquered LKS, but they have learned to live with it, to find happiness and fulfillment despite its limitations.

And so, as I prepare to close this chapter of my life

and reflect on the many stories I have been a part of, I am filled with gratitude for the lessons I have learned and the lives I have touched. I am reminded that some-times, the greatest triumphs are not the ones we see on a scan or a test result, but the ones we witness in the hearts and souls of those we care for.

In the end, the patient with LKS taught me that true healing goes beyond the physical, beyond the restoration of lost abilities. It is about finding the strength to keep going, to adapt and thrive in the face of adversity. It is about the power of love, family, and community to lift us up and carry us through even the darkest of times.

And so, as I look to the future, I carry with me the lessons learned from this remarkable patient and their family. I am inspired by their courage, their resilience, and their unwavering commitment to each other. And I am reminded that, as a doctor, my role is not just to treat the disease, but to support and empower the human spirit in its fight against all odds.

Continue with CODE BLUE: VOLUME 8

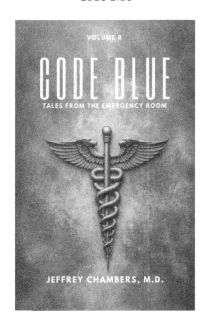

About the Author

Dr. Jeffrey Chambers is a seasoned and respected figure in the field of emergency medicine, bringing with him decades of experience and a deep well of wisdom garnered from years spent in the hectic, high-stakes environment of emergency rooms. Born and raised in Chicago, Illinois, Jeffery developed an early fascination with the intricacies of the human body and the art of healing, leading him down the path of medicine.

Earning his medical degree from the prestigious Northwestern University Feinberg School of Medicine, Dr. Chambers exhibited a natural aptitude for swift decision-making and calm demeanor under pressure, making him a perfect fit for emergency medicine. He completed his residency at the University of Chicago Medical Center, where he was exposed to a diverse range of medical emergencies, each one contributing to his growing reservoir of knowledge and expertise.

Over his illustrious career, Dr. Chambers has served in various capacities in emergency departments across the United States, from busy urban centers to smaller, rural hospitals. Each setting offered unique challenges and learning opportunities, helping him develop a holistic understanding of emergency care dynamics across different communities and healthcare systems.

A dedicated healer and lifelong learner, Dr. Chambers has not only been an active practitioner but also an educator, mentor, and author. He has nurtured the next generation of emergency medicine physicians through his teaching roles at renowned medical schools and has shared his wealth of experience through numerous publications, workshops, and conferences.

Code Blue: Tales From The Emergency Room is Dr. Chambers' foray into narrative medicine, where he amalgamates his clinical expertise with his storytelling prowess to offer readers an insider's view of the poignant, thrilling, and often heart-wrenching tales unfolding within the emergency room. Through his writing, he aims to highlight the humanity, dedication, and resilience of healthcare professionals while providing readers with a deeper understanding and appreciation of the challenges and triumphs inherent in emergency medicine.

In his personal life, Dr. Chambers is a devoted husband and father, an avid reader, and a passionate advocate for accessible and equitable healthcare for all.

His journey from a curious, science-loving child to a revered emergency medicine physician is not only a testament to his commitment and skill but also an inspiring story of service, compassion, and excellence in the field of medicine.

Also by Free Reign Publishing

10-33: TRUE TALES FROM THE THIN BLUE LINE

BEYOND THE PATH

FROM ABOVE: UFO ENCOUNTERS

WENDIGO CHRONICLES

MYSTERIES IN THE FOREST

Made in United States
Orlando, FL
05 June 2024

47552355R00107